Uveitis - Basics, Diagnosis, and Treatment

Edited by Sepehr Feizi

Published in London, United Kingdom

Uveitis - Basics, Diagnosis, and Treatment
http://dx.doi.org/10.5772/intechopen.102171
Edited by Sepehr Feizi

Contributors
Anubhav Goyal, Diego Espinosa-Heidmann, Giridhar Anantharaman, Kiana Hassanpour, Luiza M. Neves, Mahesh Gopalakrishnan, Marcela Bohn de A. Alves, Raj Kumar, Sahba Fekri, Sepehr Feizi, Sunil Kumar, Teresa E. Fowler, Vamsi Kumar Attuluri, Vineet Shah

First published in London, United Kingdom, 2024 by IntechOpen
IntechOpen is the global imprint of INTECHOPEN LIMITED, registered in England and Wales, registration number: 11086078, 167-169 Great Portland Street, London, W1W 5PF, United Kingdom

British Library Cataloguing-in-Publication Data
A catalogue record for this book is available from the British Library

Additional hard and PDF copies can be obtained from orders@intechopen.com

Uveitis - Basics, Diagnosis, and Treatment
Edited by Sepehr Feizi
p. cm.
Print ISBN 978-1-83768-595-0
Online ISBN 978-1-83768-596-7
eBook (PDF) ISBN 978-1-83768-597-4

For EU product safety concerns:
IN TECH d.o.o., Prolaz Marije Krucifikse Kozulić 3, 51000 Rijeka, Croatia,
info@intechopen.com or visit our website at intechopen.com.

Meet the editor

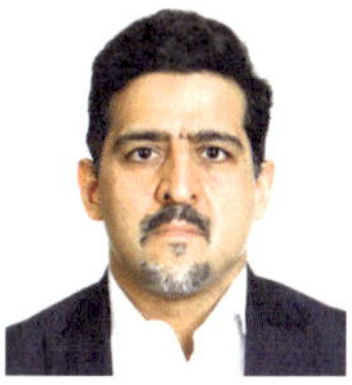

Sepehr Feizi, MD, MSc, is an experienced and highly skilled ophthalmologist with more than 20 years of experience in the field. He graduated from Islamic Azad University, Tehran, in 2000. After completing his residency in 2004 and anterior segment fellowship in 2008 at Shahid Beheshti University of Medical Sciences Tehran, he joined the Anterior Segment Service at Labbafinejad Hospital, which is affiliated with Shahid Beheshti University of Medical Sciences, Iran. He also has a master's degree in medical education. He is now an associate professor in the Department of Ophthalmology, Labbafinejad Medical Center, Iran. Dr. Feizi has published more than 150 peer-reviewed articles and 6 book chapters. He introduced, for the first time, the application of topical erythropoietin for the management of avascular conjunctival and scleral lesions.

Contents

Preface IX

Section 1
Anterior and Intermediate Uveitis 1

Chapter 1 3
Anatomy and Physiology of the Uveal Tract: Maintaining the Eye's Internal Balance
by Raj Kumar, Sunil Kumar and Vamsi Kumar Attuluri

Chapter 2 15
Herpes Simplex Virus-Associated Anterior Uveitis: Clinical Characteristics, Diagnosis, and Current Aspects on Management
by Sepehr Feizi, Sahba Fekri and Kiana Hassanpour

Chapter 3 27
Juvenile Idiopathic Arthritis-Associated Uveitis: Evidence-Based Screening, Monitoring, and Treatment
by Luiza M. Neves and Marcela Bohn de A. Alves

Section 2
Posterior Uveitis 51

Chapter 4 53
Vogt-Koyanagi-Harada Disease: Current Diagnosis and Management
by Anubhav Goyal, Vineet Shah, Giridhar Anantharaman and Mahesh Gopalakrishnan

Chapter 5 83
Malignancies Masquerading as Uveitis
by Teresa E. Fowler and Diego Espinosa-Heidmann

Preface

Uveitis is a complex condition with a variety of etiologies and clinical manifestations. Certain types are sight-threatening if undetected and undiagnosed. Previously, the etiology of many forms of uveitis were unknown, and loss of visual acuity was frequently encountered in patients with uveitis. Over the past decade, we have come to understand the mechanisms by which the immune system results in uveitis. In addition, newly introduced technologies such as optical coherence tomography (OCT) and polymerase chain reaction (PCR) are changing the way we diagnose the underlying etiologies of uveitis. The accuracy of PCR has enabled us to diagnose infectious causes of uveitis. OCT is useful in evaluating ocular inflammation and in monitoring the response to treatment.

Treatment for uveitis was very limited before 1950. Many physicians treated these patients by inducing hyperpyrexia, in which the patients' temperatures were increased to 40° C to 41° C by placing them in steam baths for up to six hours. Although occasionally successful, this treatment could result in death. The revolution in the treatment of autoimmune diseases occurred in 1949 when corticosteroids were introduced for the management of rheumatoid arthritis. Ophthalmologists rapidly took this advantage to treat ocular inflammatory diseases with corticosteroids, which remain the mainstay therapy of uveitis. Long-standing application of corticosteroids, however, can result in serious ocular side effects such as corneal ulcers, cataracts, and glaucoma. Newly developed immunosuppressive drugs used in organ transplant surgery have helped ophthalmologists in the treatment of uveitis. In addition, we increased our knowledge of how modulating the immune response can improve clinical outcomes. Agents that specifically target cytokines and their receptors are now routinely used in the treatment of severe uveitis that is resistant to conventional treatment. Intravitreal injections and sustained-released intravitreal implants have been increasingly used by ophthalmologists to deliver high amounts of drugs to target tissues in the eyes while avoiding systemic adverse reactions.

This book provides both a practical approach to the diagnosis and management of different types of uveitis. The book is categorized into two sections. Section 1 consists of three chapters: "Anatomy and Physiology of the Uveal Tract: Maintaining the Eye's Internal Balance", "Herpes Simplex Virus-Associated Anterior Uveitis: Clinical Characteristics, Diagnosis, and Current Aspects on Management", and "Juvenile Idiopathic Arthritis-Associated Uveitis: Evidence-Based Screening, Monitoring, and Treatment". Section 2 discusses the etiologies of panuveitis and includes the chapters: "Vogt-Koyanagi-Harada Disease: Current Diagnosis and Management" and

"Malignancies Masquerading as Uveitis". I hope that this book will be valuable to both ophthalmologists and other specialists, including rheumatologists, internists, and researchers in the field of ocular inflammatory diseases.

Sepehr Feizi, MD, MSc
Ocular Tissue Engineering Research Center,
Research Institute for Ophthalmology and Vision Science,
Shahid Beheshti University of Medical Sciences,
Tehran, Iran

Section 1

Anterior and Intermediate Uveitis

Chapter 1

Anatomy and Physiology of the Uveal Tract: Maintaining the Eye's Internal Balance

Raj Kumar, Sunil Kumar and Vamsi Kumar Attuluri

Abstract

The uveal tract, comprising the iris, ciliary body, and choroid, is pivotal in maintaining the eye's internal balance. The iris, with its pigmentation, regulates light entry through pupil control and contributes to eye color variation. The ciliary body, positioned behind the iris, facilitates accommodation by adjusting the lens for focusing at various distances and produces aqueous humor, crucial for intraocular pressure maintenance. The choroid, a vascular layer at the back of the eye, nourishes the retina. Together, these components uphold eye shape, control light entry, and support retinal function. Understanding uveal anatomy and physiology is fundamental to comprehending ocular mechanisms, encompassing both structural integrity and functional dynamics. This book chapter provides a knowledge of uveal anatomy and physiology.

Keywords: uveal tract, ciliary body, iris, choroid tissue, aqueous humor, anterior segment, sclera, retina

1. Introduction

The uveal tract, encompassing the iris, ciliary body, and choroid, is integral to maintaining the delicate internal equilibrium of the eye. These components work synergistically to regulate light entry, support retinal function, and sustain intraocular pressure. Understanding the intricate anatomy and physiological interactions within the uveal tract is essential for comprehending the complexities of ocular health and vision. In this chapter, we delve into the detailed anatomy and dynamic physiology of the uveal tract, shedding light on its crucial role in preserving the eye's internal balance and functionality (**Figure 1**) [1].

The ciliary body produces aqueous humor, a clear fluid that fills the front part of the eye and helps to maintain the eye's shape and pressure [2]. The choroid is a layer of blood vessels that provides oxygen and nutrients to the retina [3]. Together, these structures help to maintain the eye's overall health and function (**Figure 2**) [4].

1.1 Iris

The iris is the colored part of the eye that surrounds the pupil, which controls the amount of light that enters the eye. It is responsible for regulating the size of the

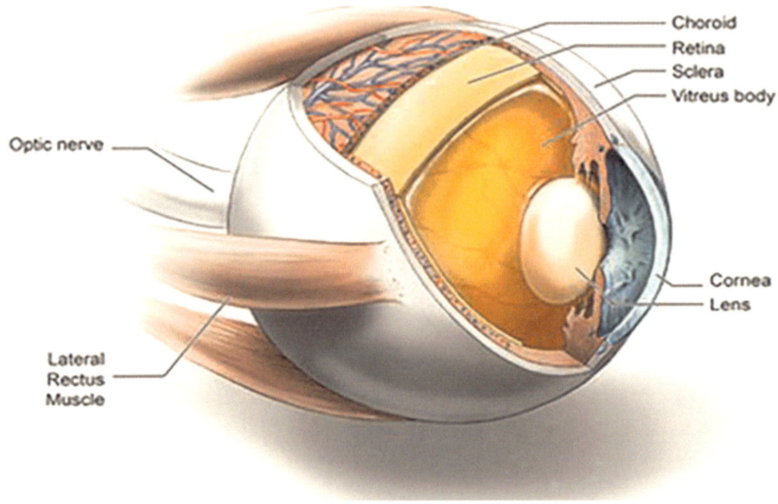

Figure 1.
The uveal tract consists of three parts: Iris, ciliary body and choroid. Adapted from the public domain, https://www.nih.gov/news-events/news-releases/eyes-cjd-patients-show-evidence-prions. Credit: Ryan Kissinger, NIAID.

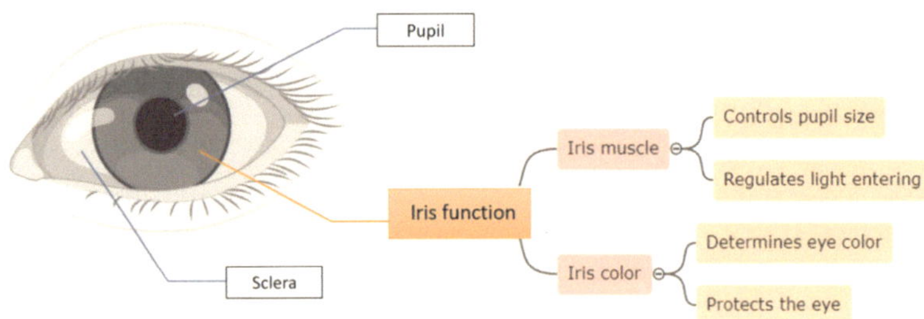

Figure 2.
Functions of iris (anterior most part of uveal tract). Created with the help of BioRender.com.

pupil and the amount of light that enters the eye. In humans, the iris is typically brown, blue, green, or hazel in color [3, 5]. The iris also contains a ring-shaped muscle called the sphincter pupillae, which constricts the pupil in response to bright light, and a muscle called the dilator pupillae, which dilates the pupil in dim light. Some eye diseases and conditions can affect the iris, such as iritis (inflammation of the iris) and heterochromia (difference in color between the irises) (**Figure 3**) [6].

(Anterior most part of uveal tract)
Thin circular disc.
Average diameter 12 mm.
Thickness 0.5 mm.
Center *aperture* 3–4 mm known as *Pupil.*
Pupil regulates the amount of light entering the eye [2].

DOI: http://dx.doi.org/10.5772/intechopen.114947

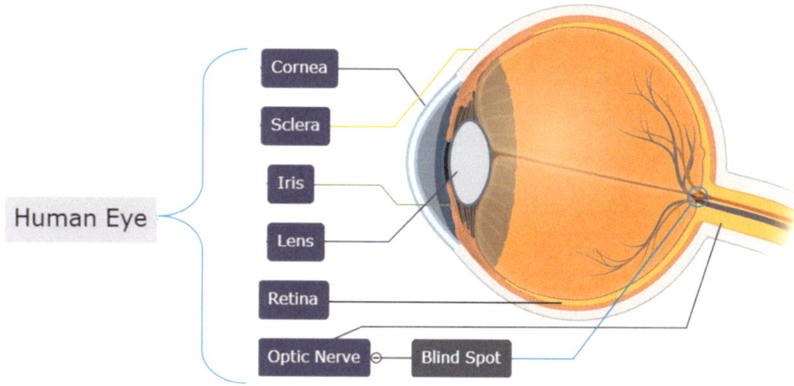

Figure 3.
Parts of human eye image. Created with the help of BioRender.com.

1.1.1 Macroscopic appearance

1.1.1.1 Anterior surface

- Divided into ciliary and pupiallary
- Zone by a zigzag line *collarette*

1.1.1.2 Ciliary zone

- Radial streaks
- Straight when pupil dilated
- Wavy when pupil constricted
- Due to underlying *radial vessels*

1.1.1.3 Crypts

- Depressions where superficial layer of iris is missing
- Two rows Peripheral Iris root
- Central near Collarette

1.1.1.4 Contraction furrows

- Faint lines concentric to Collarette more marked on outer part of ciliary zone
- More prominent when pupil dilates.

1.1.1.5 Pupillary zone

- 1.6 mm wide
- Between collarette and pigmented papillary frill.
- Relatively smooth and flat

1.1.1.6 Pupillary frill

- Fringe of black pigment at Pupillary margin
- Due to slight extension of posterior pigment epithelium of iris round the edge of pupil

1.1.1.7 Posterior surface

- Dark brown or black
- Broken by furrows only
- Those near papillary margin are known as *Schwalbe's contraction folds*
- Those which run downwards between the ciliary processes are known as *Schwalbe's structural folds* besides several circular furrows [7].

1.2 Microscopic structure of iris

The iris is made up of two main layers: the anterior part of iris is stroma and the posterior part is iris pigment epithelium. The pigmented epithelium is a thin layer of cells that contains melanin, the pigment that gives the iris its color. The stroma is the thicker, more complex layer of the iris that gives it its shape. It is made up of fibroblasts, a type of cell that produces collagen and other fibers, as well as blood vessels and nerves [8].

The stroma of the iris also contains muscle fibers that make up the sphincter pupillae and dilator pupillae, which control the size of the pupil [9]. The iris also contains the crypts of the iris, which are small, deep recesses in the stroma that are thought to help protect the eye from injury by diverting debris away from the pupil. Overall, the iris is a complex and important part of the eye that plays a crucial role in regulating the amount of light that enters the eye and helping the eye to see clearly [1, 10].

Layers:

1. Anterior limiting layer
2. Stroma
3. Anterior pigmented epithelial layer
4. Posterior pigmented epithelial layer

5. Anterior limiting layer

    - Condensation of anterior part of stroma
    - Deficient at crypts, thin at contraction furrows
    - The type and density of pigment in this layer gives definitive color to iris
        - Blue iris—this layer is thin and has few pigmented cells
        - Brown Iris—thick and doubly pigmented [9]

6. Stroma

    - Main bulk of iris loose connective tissue
    - Contains
        - Pupil constrictor muscle
        - Pupil dilator muscle
        - Vessels nerves and pigment cells
        - Other cells lymphocytes, fibroblasts, macrophages etc.

1.2.1 Pupil constrictor muscle

- 1 mm broad band in pupillary part
- Flat circular band of plain muscle fibers
- Nerve supply parasympathetic fibers through third nerve
- Constrics the pupil

1.2.2 Pupil dilator muscle

- Present in posterior part of stroma of ciliary zone
- Nerve supply cervical sympathetic
- Dilates the pupil

1.2.3 Blood vessels

- Main bulk of stroma
- Branches from major arterial circle

- Responsible for radial streaks on anterior surface
- Straight when pupil constricts
- Wavy when pupil dilates
- Pigment cells melanocytes—branched} Clump cells—circular} both contain melanin [9].

1. Anterior epithelial layer
    - Gives rise to dilator pupillae
2. Posterior pigmented epithelial layer
    - It forms papillary frill at pupillary margin
    - Pigment cells are columnar type contain dark brown pigment granules.

1.3 Ciliary body

The ciliary body is a ring-shaped structure located in the eye, between the iris and the choroid. It plays an important role in maintaining the shape of the eye's lens. The ciliary body also contains the ciliary muscle, which is responsible for changing the shape of the lens in order to adjust the eye's focal length. This process is called accommodation and allows the eye to focus on objects at different distances. The ciliary body also produces aqueous humor, a clear fluid that nourishes the eye and helps to maintain its shape [11].

Ciliary body begins at ora serrata when choroid and retina ends (**Figure 4**).

Easily recognized by its black color (Whereas choroid is brown).

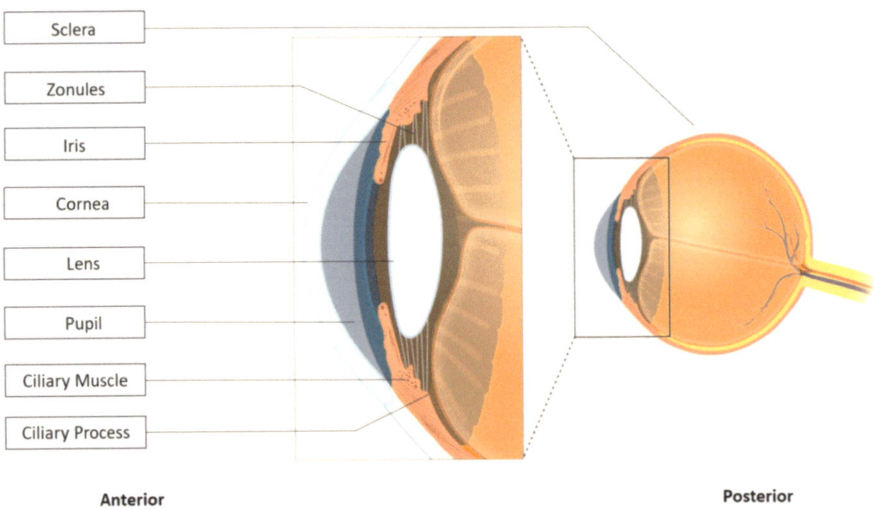

Figure 4.
Anterior cross section of the human eye (ciliary body). Created with the help of BioRender.com.

Symmetrical girdle, narrow above and nasally and broader below and temporally.
Triangular Apex continuous with choroid.
Base toward cornea.
Externally sclera.
Internally vitreous body.
Smooth near ora pars plana.
Finger like processes near base (anteriorly).

1.4 Microscopic structure

The ciliary body is a ring-shaped structure located behind the iris in the eye. It is composed of both muscle and glandular tissue. The ciliary muscle is responsible for controlling the shape of the lens, which helps to focus light on the retina. The ciliary body also contains the ciliary epithelium, which produces aqueous humor, a clear fluid that fills the front chamber of the eye and helps to nourish and maintain the shape of the lens and cornea [12]. Following are the main points to be remembered while studying the microscopic structure.

1.4.1 Supra ciliary lamina

- Outermost condensed part of stroma,
- Consists of collagen fibers (pigmented)
- Posteriorly continuous with suprachoroidal lamina
- Anteriorly continuous with anterior limiting membrane of iris

1.4.2 Stroma of ciliary body

- Consists of collagen and fibrblasts
- Contains

1.4.2.1 Ciliary muscle

Non striated, occupies outer part of ciliary body [13].

1.4.2.1.1 Three parts

- Longitudinal fibers—Origin sclera spur insertion suprachoroidal lamina
- Circular fibers—Present anteriorly and in inner portion and run parallel to limbus (Lies nearest to lens)
- Radial fibers—Obliquely placed fibers which continuous with circular fibers.
- Action—To slacken the suspensory ligament of lens and thus help in accommodation.

1.4.2.2 Vascular stroma of ciliary body

- Major arterial circle lies just anterior to circular muscle fibers
- Formed by anastomosis between long posterior ciliary arteries and anterior ciliary arteries
- Send branches to iris and ciliary body

2. Layer of pigmented epithelium

- Forward continuation of retinal pigment epithelium continues as anterior pigment epithelium of iris

3. Layer of non pigmented epithelium

- Forward continuation of sensory retina which stops at ora serrata. Continues as posterior pigment epithelium of iris

4. Internal limiting membranes

- Lines non pigmented epithelium and is forward continuation of internal limiting membrane of retina [14].

4.1 Ciliary processes

- Site of aqueous production
- Whitish finger like projection from pars plicata of ciliary body
- Number 70–80 Size 2 × 0.5 mm

4.2 Choroid

The choroid is a layer of tissue located in the eye between the retina and the sclera (the white of the eye). It contains blood vessels that provide oxygen and nutrients to the retina, as well as pigment cells that help to absorb light and reduce glare. Damage or disease of the choroid can lead to vision problems (**Figure 5**).

- Posterior part of vascular coat
- Extends from optic disc to ora
- Inner surface smooth, brown lies in contact with pigment epithelium of retina
- Outer surface rough in contact with sclera thicker
- Posteriorly (0.22) compared to Anteriorly (0.1)

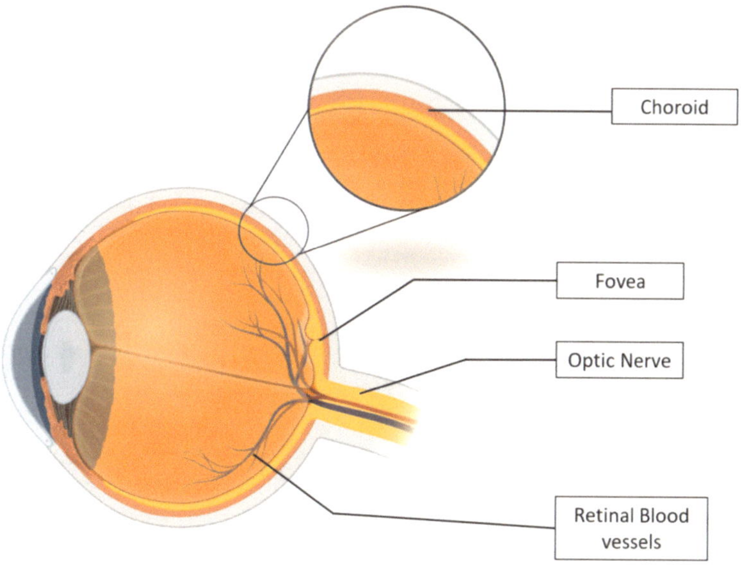

Figure 5.
Choroid. Created with the help of BioRender.com.

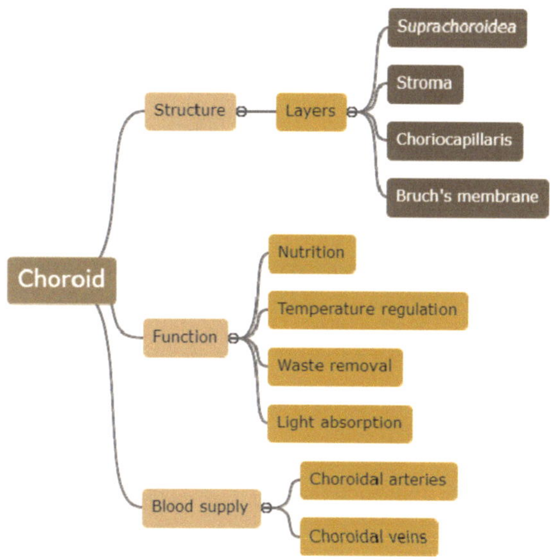

Figure 6.
Microscopic structure of the choroid.

Microscopic Structure Explained with flow chart (See **Figure 6**).

1. Supra choroidal lamina thin membrane of condensed collagen continuous anteriorly with supraciliary lamina.

   Space between this and sclera-supra choroidal space contains long ciliary and short posterior ciliary arteries.

2. Strom mainly formed by vessels arranged in two layers

Outer large Haller's layer.

Inner medium Sattler's layer.

Also cells pigment cells, macrophages mast cells plasma cells

3. Choriocapillaris: Rich capillary network, Gets most of the blood from medium and large vessels from stroma. Nourishes pigment epithelium and outer layers of sensory retina.

4. Basal lamina (Bruch's membrane)

   Multi-layered structure lies between choriocapillaris and pigment epithelium of retina becomes thickened with age and produces hyaline excrescence known as drusens.

5. Conclusion

The present chapter was written to understand the detailed anatomy and the Microscopic examination of the eye's Uveal region along with its structure and functions. This chapter will be good direction for the Graduate, Master and clinical optometry course students and will be a good note and reading material during the examinations and interview preparation for competitive exams as well as jobs.

Acknowledgements

I would like to thanks my PhD Guide Sr. Professor A.K. Khurana, Ex. PGI Rohtak for motivating us for to write the book chapter, for his continuous motivation for writing this book chapter, Authors are also thankful to Galgotias University for providing the basic amenities and affiliation. We are also thankful to the authors and the public domains whose images are used and the link are pasted just below the image.

We are also thankful to the Ken Pekoc (NIH/NIAID) for giving us permission for the use of image in our book chapter.

Notes

Figure 1 is adapted from the (NIH/NIAID) with author's permission, **Figure 2**, **Figure 3**, **Figure 4** **Figure 5** and **Figure 6** created with the help of biorender.com. Mr. Vamsi Kumar Attuluri created all the images for this book chapter.

Author details

Raj Kumar[1*], Sunil Kumar[2*] and Vamsi Kumar Attuluri[3]

1 Department of Optometry, School of Allied and Health Sciences, Galgotias University, Greater Noida, India

2 Department of Clinical Embryology and Reproductive Genetics, (Origin LIFE) Rayat Bahra University, India

3 Department of Medical Lab Technology, Chandigarh University, Mohali, Punjab, India

*Address all correspondence to: raj@galgotiasuniversity.edu.in, optomrajlvpei@gmail.com and skjaswalmicro085@gmail.com

References

[1] James DG. Multi-system ocular syndromes. Journal of the Royal College of Physicians of London. 1974;**9**(1):63

[2] Miller PE. Uvea. Slatter's Fundamentals of Veterinary Ophthalmology. 2008:203-229. DOI: 10.1016/B978-072160561-6.50014-9. [Epub 2009 June 5]. PMCID: PMC714 9650

[3] Pavan-Langston D, Galor A, Perez VL. Uveal tract: Iris, ciliary body, and choroid. In: Man of Ocular Diagnosis Therapy. 3rd ed. Little Boston: Brown Co.; 1991. pp. 173-218

[4] Ludwig M, Garden AS, Williams MD, Gombos DS. Management of uveal melanoma. In: Esmaeli B, editor. Ophthalmic Oncology. M.D. Anderson Solid Tumor Oncology Series. Vol. 6. Boston, MA: Springer; 2010. DOI: 10.1007/978-1-4419-0374-7_15

[5] Pavan-Langston D, Galor A, Perez VL. Uveal tract: Iris, ciliary body, and choroid. In: Mannis MJ, Macsai MS, editors. Eye and Contact Lens: Research, Clinical, and Experimental. 3rd ed. Boston: Lippincott Williams & Wilkins; 2019. pp. 173-218

[6] Collaborative Ocular Melanoma Study Group. Histopathologic characteristics of uveal melanomas in eyes enucleated from the collaborative ocular melanoma study COMS report no. 6. American Journal of Ophthalmology. 1998;**125**(6):745-766

[7] Ramasamy A, Harrisson SE, Clasper JC, Stewart MPM. Injuries from roadside improvised explosive devices. The Journal of Trauma: Injury, Infection, and Critical Care. 2008;**65**(4):910-914. DOI: 10.1097/TA.0b013e3181848cf6

[8] Skalicky SE, Skalicky SE. The ciliary body and aqueous fluid formation and drainage. Ocular and Visual Physiology: Clinical Application. 2016;**1**:67-83

[9] Shields CL, Welch RJ, Malik K, Acaba-Berrocal LA, Selzer EB, Newman JH, et al. Uveal metastasis: Clinical features and survival outcome of 2214 tumors in 1111 patients based on primary tumor origin. Middle East African Journal of Ophthalmology. 2018;**25**(2):81-90. DOI: 10.4103/meajo.MEAJO_6_18. PMID: 30122853; PMCID: PMC6071342

[10] Gupta N, Motlagh M, Singh G. Anatomy, Head and Neck, Eye Arteries. 2019

[11] McMenamin PG. The distribution of immune cells in the uveal tract of the normal eye. Eye. 1997;**11**(2):183-193

[12] Pang CE et al. Ultra-widefield imaging with autofluorescence and indocyanine green angiography in central serous chorioretinopathy. American Journal of Ophthalmology. 2014;**158**(2):362-371

[13] Sayan M et al. Clinical management of uveal melanoma: A comprehensive review with a treatment algorithm. Radiation Oncology Journal. 2020;**38**(3): 162

[14] Ofri R. Development and congenital abnormalities. In: Maggs DJ, Miller PE, Ofri R, editors. Slatter's Fundamentals of Veterinary Ophthalmology. Vol. 4. 2007. pp. 20-32

Chapter 2

Herpes Simplex Virus-Associated Anterior Uveitis: Clinical Characteristics, Diagnosis, and Current Aspects on Management

Sepehr Feizi, Sahba Fekri and Kiana Hassanpour

Abstract

Herpes simplex virus (HSV)-associated anterior uveitis accounts for 5–10% of patients with anterior uveitis and 3–10% of all uveitis patients, and is the most frequent etiology of infectious anterior uveitis. It is chiefly an acute unilateral iritis involving middle-aged individuals with preponderance in females. The clinical features of HSV anterior uveitis may mimic other non-infectious and infectious anterior uveitis entities, particularly at the early stage of the disease. Confirmed prior HSV infection and the presence of characteristic ocular findings such as keratitis, high intraocular pressure, and sectoral or patchy iris atrophy suggest the diagnosis and help to differentiate this condition from other etiologies of anterior uveitis. New diagnostic techniques, including evaluation of intraocular fluids applying polymerase chain reaction for viral DNA and the Goldmann–Witmer coefficient for antibodies against the virus can confirm the diagnosis in cases with no specific signs of HSV anterior uveitis. Oral antivirals and topical corticosteroids have become the main standards for treatment.

Keywords: herpes simplex virus, anterior uveitis, immunopathology, clinical characteristics, differential diagnosis, laboratory tests, treatment

1. Introduction

The majority of acute iritis cases are either associated with HLA-B27 positivity or idiopathic. Herpes simplex virus (HSV) uveitis accounts for 5–10% of patients with anterior uveitis and 3–10% of all uveitis patients and is the most frequent etiology of infectious anterior uveitis [1]. This entity is an acute unilateral uveitis chiefly involving middle-aged immunocompetent individuals with preponderance in females. However, several bilateral HSV anterior uveitis cases have been described, often in immunocompromised patients [2].

HSV anterior uveitis can be easily diagnosed in the background of confirmed prior HSV ocular disease, typical herpetic dermatitis, dendritic keratitis, or iris atrophy, but these findings are often absent at first presentation [3]. In such situations, the diagnosis requires a high index of clinical suspicion and is based on clinical characteristics, including corneal opacity, decreased corneal sensation, and acutely increased intraocular pressure [3]. Other infectious agents of anterior uveitis including varicella zoster virus (VZV) and cytomegalovirus (CMV) can be associated with keratic precipitates (KPs), high intraocular pressure, and sectoral or patchy iris atrophy [4, 5]. Therefore, it is crucial to ask patients about previous diseases, general health, and the onset of the disease. In addition, they should be evaluated for non-infectious etiologies including sarcoidosis and HLA-B27 phenotype. Acute anterior uveitis caused by noninfectious etiologies tends to alternate between eyes. Recurrent episodes of anterior uveitis in the same eye should alert the ophthalmologist to consider herpetic etiology, even though most episodes of recurrent anterior uveitis confined to one eye are not caused by HSV in origin [3].

The gold standard diagnostic technique for HSV anterior uveitis is the detection of the viral genome or elevated concentrations of anti-viral antibodies in aqueous humor. However, these tests are not accessible to all ophthalmologists, and clinical diagnosis allows to start of appropriate treatment before the results of the molecular evaluation of aqueous humor are identified [6]. Oral antivirals and topical corticosteroids have become the main standards for treatment. In this chapter, we review the immunopathology, clinical findings, differential diagnoses, laboratory tests, and treatment modalities in HSV anterior uveitis. In addition, we describe the long-term prognosis and future directions for the management of the disease.

2. Immunopathology of HSV anterior uveitis

The majority of cases of ocular herpes infection are caused by HSV type 1 [7]. The primary infection which can be asymptomatic typically occurs during early childhood [7]. The virus establishes a ganglionic latency in the trigeminal nerve and lies dormant until triggered to proliferate, migrate down nerves, and establish recurrent infection in the area supplied by that nerve [7]. Despite the vast majority of the general population being latently infected with HSV type 1, only a few individuals develop anterior uveitis. Several factors influence the rate and type of ocular herpetic diseases, including age, genetic predisposition, immune status, virus strain, and route of infection [8, 9]. Both innate and adaptive immunity are essential to prevent HSV-1 reactivation [10]. Failure of this immune control results in the reactivation of the latent virus and may result in different ocular herpetic diseases such as anterior uveitis [7]. Left or right trigeminal ganglion is involved independently by latent HSV which explains the clinical observation that HSV anterior uveitis is usually unilateral [11, 12].

The pathogenesis of HSV anterior uveitis is believed to involve a cytopathic effect of the actively replicating pathogen on ocular tissue during the early phase and the host immune responses during the late phase of the disease [7]. The genetic makeup of patients, their immune status, and the characteristics of the virus determine the severity and outcome of the resulting uveitis. HSV causes an acute lytic infection which results in the release of different inflammatory chemokines and cytokines [7]. This innate immune response attracts immune cells, predominantly CD 8+ T cells. The aqueous humor of HSV anterior uveitis patients is typically devoid of neutrophils [7]. T cells secret more chemokines and cytokines, including interferon gamma and tumor necrosis factor alpha, and apply cytotoxicity toward the virus-infected cells which further exacerbates the inflammation [13]. High intraocular pressure encountered during the acute phase of HSV anterior uveitis is a local inflammatory response rather than the viral cytopathic effect on the trabecular meshwork. This hypothesis is confirmed by the beneficial effect of corticosteroid treatment on high intraocular pressure [5]. Chronic application of corticosteroid eye drops and trabecular meshwork damage owing to long-term and recurrent inflammation can result in a permanent elevation in intraocular pressure in a subset of affected individuals.

3. Clinical findings

Each episode of HSV anterior uveitis is characterized by decreased visual acuity, redness, pain, and photophobia. The episodes may last from several days to several months and tend to recur once per year, on average. Clinical findings include herpetic dermatoblepharitis (blisters), conjunctivitis, keratitis, iritis, and retinitis [5].

3.1 Corneal involvement

Corneal involvement which is present in 30–40% of patients with HSV anterior uveitis includes epithelial keratitis, disciform keratitis, active interstitial keratitis, endotheliitis, corneal edema, and old opacities (**Figures 1–3**) [5]. Dendritic keratitis is transient and generally presents less frequently during recurrent disease, especially at uveitis onset. Corneal edema can result from interstitial keratitis and endotheliitis but may also be secondary to episodes of increased intraocular pressure [5]. Many patients also have decreased corneal sensation [5].

3.2 Anterior uveitis

The iritis can be nongranulomatous but is more frequently granulomatous with moderate size mutton fat KPs, usually in a triangular shape [4]. KPs can be situated

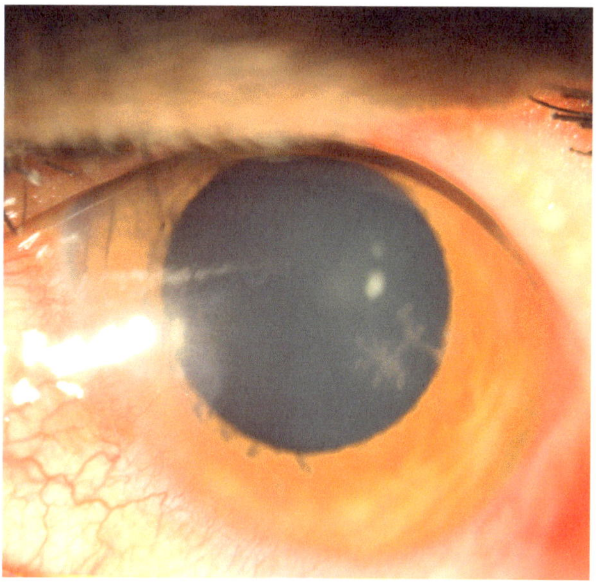

Figure 1.
Diffuse slit-lamp photograph demonstrates epithelial keratitis in an eye with herpes simplex virus-associated anterior uveitis. The dendritic lesion has a branching pattern and terminal end bulbs.

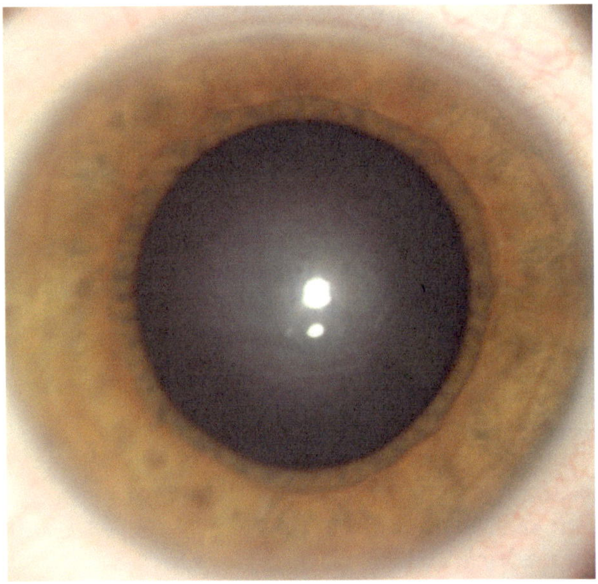

Figure 2.
Diffuse slit-lamp photograph demonstrates herpes simplex virus disciform keratitis. The lesion is characterized by corneal stromal edema with folds in the Descemet membrane. There is no active infiltration in the corneal stroma.

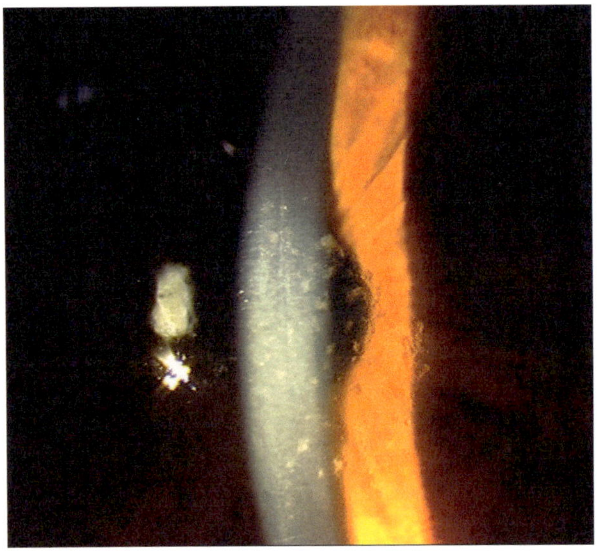

Figure 3.
Corneal involvement in herpes simplex virus-associated anterior uveitis. Diffuse slit-lamp photograph demonstrates stromal infiltration and edema with small to medium size keratic precipitates under the area of active corneal involvement.

inferiorly; however, they collect frequently under the area of active corneal involvement (**Figure 3**). Anterior chamber inflammation may vary from mild to severe and can be associated with hypopyon or hyphema.

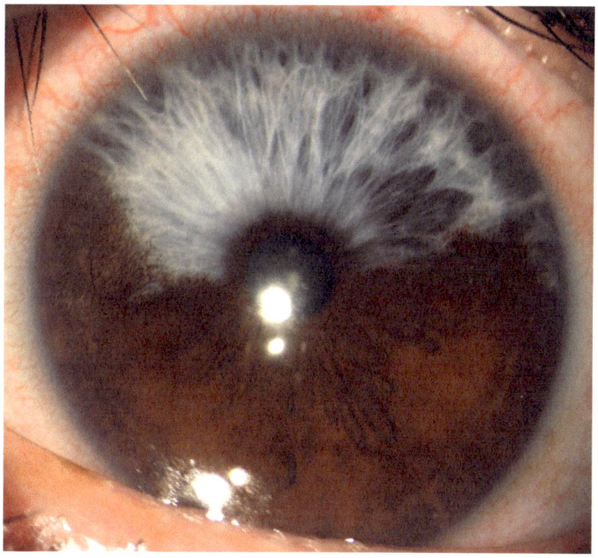

Figure 4.
Sectoral iris atrophy in an eye with previous episodes of herpes simplex virus-associated anterior uveitis.

3.3 High intraocular pressure

High intraocular pressure (>30 mmHg) is encountered in 46–90% of the cases; this highlights the importance of close observation of intraocular pressure in HSV anterior uveitis [4, 14, 15]. Elevated intraocular pressure usually rapidly decreases following the administration of topical corticosteroids and anti-glaucoma medication. However, a minority of these patients (18–31%) may progress to secondary glaucoma, necessitating long-term application of anti-glaucoma medication or a filtering procedure [4, 5, 14, 16, 17].

3.4 Iris abnormalities

Ischemic necrosis of the iris stroma leads to iris atrophy that is characterized by a well-defined defect involving iris stroma and pigment epithelium. Typical for HSV anterior uveitis is patchy or sectoral iris atrophy (**Figure 4**); however, diffuse iris atrophy may develop due to different pathological mechanisms such as inflammation [5, 14]. Iris atrophy is best seen on retroillumination and may distort the pupil. It is a very valuable sign for the diagnosis of HSV anterior uveitis [14]. This sign, however, is usually absent during the acute phase of the disease. Therefore, iris atrophy is only a helpful diagnostic criterion in chronic or recurrent forms of the disease [14]. Posterior synechiae are another iris abnormality which are seen in 50% of the affected patients [4].

4. Differential diagnosis

The clinical presentations of HSV anterior uveitis can be seen in other infectious and non-infectious anterior uveitis cases particularly at the early stage [4, 5].

However, some subtle differences may be helpful in distinguishing anterior uveitis caused by HSV from other viral etiologies, including VZV and CMV, and non-infectious etiologies [18].

4.1 VZV anterior uveitis

Anterior uveitis caused by VZV occurs in older individuals (60 years) than HSV anterior uveitis (50 years), however, the age distributions overlap [5, 14, 18]. A history of ipsilateral zoster dermatitis is useful in the diagnosis of VZV-associated anterior uveitis, but dermatomal zoster is not always present [5]. Keratitis is less frequent in cases with VZV anterior uveitis (<3%) compared to cases with HSV anterior uveitis [5]. The pattern of dendritic epithelial lesions, when present, is helpful in differentiating HSV from VZV as the etiology of anterior uveitis. HSV dendrites demonstrate a branching pattern, with fluorescein staining in the ulcer base, rose bengal staining at the border, and terminal end bulbs (**Figure 1**). In contrast, VZV pseudodendrites are frequently broader, polymorphous, and slightly elevated, with few terminal dilatations, less regular branching, and no ulceration (**Figure 5**). Severe and diffuse reduction in corneal sensation favors the diagnosis of VZV uveitis, but corneal sensation can be profoundly decreased by HSV as well [5]. The intensity of anterior chamber reaction is higher in VZV than in HSV anterior uveitis, whereas fibrin formation in the anterior chamber has been reported less frequently in VZV (5%) than in HSV (13%) associated anterior uveitis [5]. The incidence of elevated intraocular pressure has been reported in 63% of cases with HSV anterior uveitis and 85% of cases with VZV anterior uveitis with a higher intraocular pressure level observed in VZV infection [5]. Sectoral or patchy iris atrophy and posterior iris synechiae are equally encountered in these two etiologies of anterior uveitis [5, 18].

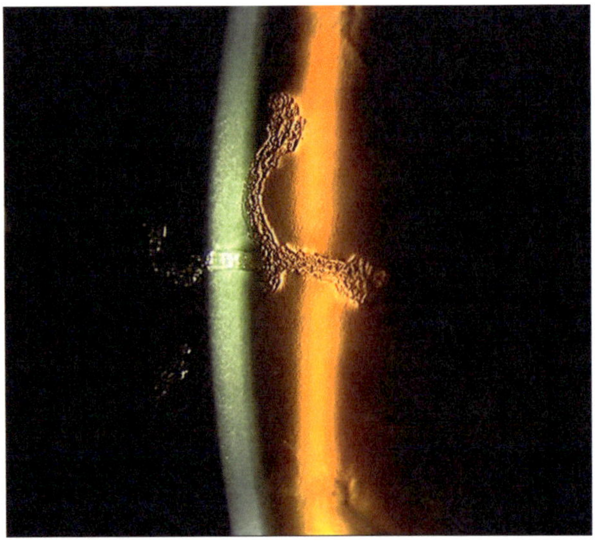

Figure 5.
Diffuse slit-lamp photograph demonstrates a pseudodendrite in an eye with varicella zoster virus-associated anterior uveitis. The pseudodendrite is characterized by its broad, polymorphous, and slightly elevated appearance, with few terminal dilatations, less regular branching, and no ulceration.

4.2 CMV anterior uveitis

CMV has recently implicated in acute, recurrent, or chronic iritis in patients with the competent immune system. Several clues can differentiate this entity from HSV anterior uveitis. Endotheliitis is less common in CMV than HSV anterior uveitis, however, coin-shaped nodular KPs and reduced endothelial cell count reported in CMV anterior uveitis are not associated with HSV anterior uveitis [5]. Medium size KPs are more frequently seen in HSV anterior uveitis than CMV anterior uveitis which tends to have fine to small size KPs [4, 5]. Eyes with CMV anterior uveitis have no corneal opacities, and iris transillumination, when present, is patchy rather than sectoral as seen in HSV uveitis [5]. Moreover, anterior chamber reaction is less severe and fibrin formation has not been reported in CMV anterior uveitis [5]. Posterior iris synechiae is frequent in HSV uveitis but absent in CMV anterior uveitis, whereas peripheral anterior synechiae is more frequent in the latter [5]. Nodule formation at trabecular meshwork by gonioscopic examination is less frequently observed in CMV than in HSV anterior uveitis (6 vs. 13%, respectively) [5]. The incidence of elevated intraocular pressure has been reported in 78% of eyes with CMV anterior uveitis, and intractable glaucoma develops more frequently in CMV anterior uveitis compared to HSV uveitis [5, 19]. Finally, CMV should be considered in cases who are diagnosed with HSV anterior uveitis but fail to respond to acyclovir and corticosteroids.

4.3 Fuchs' heterochromic iridocyclitis

It can be challenging to differentiate Fuchs' heterochromic iridocyclitis from HSV anterior uveitis as both entities can demonstrate fine stellate KPs, high intraocular pressure, and iris atrophy. In Fuchs' uveitis syndrome, however, KPs are fine, feathery, and diffuse, and diffuse stromal atrophy results in loss of the corrugated appearance of the iris. Moreover, transillumination defects are radial rather than patchy or sectoral. High intraocular pressure in Fuchs' heterochromic iridocyclitis is unresponsive to topical corticosteroids and antiviral medication as it is caused by damage to the trabecular meshwork rather than a transient inflammation. In addition, posterior synechiae are not the feature. Other specific findings in Fuchs' heterochromic iridocyclitis include heterochromia and small translucent nodules at the pupil border. Recently, some investigators have suggested that Fuchs' uveitis syndrome may be caused by CMV and rubella virus.

4.4 Posner-Schlossman syndrome (glaucomatocyclitic crisis)

The Posner-Schlossman syndrome is characterized by fine and medium size KPs either in a linear or ring pattern, mild to moderate anterior chamber reaction, and an acute increase in intraocular pressure. Patchy or diffuse iris atrophy is common. It has been suggested that this syndrome may have an association with HSV infection; Van der Lelij et al. [14] found that approximately 20% of the cases with HSV anterior uveitis were initially diagnosed with Posner-Schlossman syndrome [14].

5. Laboratory test

The diagnosis of HSV anterior uveitis can be confirmed by analyzing aqueous humor for the virus genome and antibodies against virus antigens. Polymerase chain reaction (PCR) for viral DNA had a sensitivity and specificity of 91.3 and 98.8%, respectively [20]. A less commonly used technique is the Goldmann-Witmer coefficient (GWC), which measures the level of anti-herpes antibodies in aqueous humor. The GWC compares the ratio of antibodies directed against the virus in serum and aqueous humor with that of total immunoglobulin G in serum and aqueous humor; a ratio > 3 is considered positive. This test is less specific than PCR because anti-HSV antibodies can cross-react with antibodies directed against VZV [4, 14]. In addition, the results of the GWC may vary depending on the duration of the uveitis; the viral genome is readily detectable, and local antibody is absent at the onset of the disease, whereas the reverse result is more frequent when aqueous humor is sampled later [21]. Moreover, the GWC is more helpful when the patient's immune system is normal, and false-negative result has been reported in severely immunocompromised patients [21, 22]. For these reasons, both PCR and GWC should preferably be performed simultaneously.

6. Treatment

Oral antivirals and topical corticosteroids have become the mainstays of treatment to reduce virus replication and T cell-mediated response against viral antigens, respectively. Other medications prescribed for the treatment of HSV anterior uveitis include cycloplegic and ocular antihypertensive agents [23].

6.1 Antiviral treatment

Several antiviral agents are currently available for the treatment of HSV anterior uveitis. Oral acyclovir, 400 mg five times a day, is reported to provide adequate concentrations in tears and aqueous humor, essentially eradicating the need for topical antiviral medication, even in eyes with active keratitis. Oral acyclovir can reduce the duration of HSV-induced inflammation as well as the chance of recurrent epithelial lesions with topical corticosteroids. Maintenance doses of oral acyclovir, 400 mg twice a day, when prescribed on a long-term basis (more than 6 months) have been demonstrated to reduce the recurrent episodes of HSV anterior uveitis.

Similar antiviral effects have been shown with oral valacyclovir, 1 g three times a day and famciclovir, 500 mg three times a day for 1 week, while providing the advantage of convenient dosing. Compared to oral acyclovir, oral valacyclovir, a pro-drug of acyclovir, is absorbed more efficiently and provides threefold to fourfold higher blood concentration. Valacyclovir should probably be avoided in patients infected by the human immunodeficiency virus as this drug can cause the thrombocytopenic purpura/hemolytic uremic syndrome in these cases [23].

The majority of topical antiviral agents do not reach therapeutic levels in the aqueous humor and can cause corneal epitheliopathy or allergic blepharoconjunctivitis in 5–10% of patients with long-term use [23]. The only exception is acyclovir ointment which is usually well tolerated, even with prolonged use, and has good ocular penetration providing adequate concentrations in aqueous humor. Therefore, acyclovir ointment 3% four times a day can be administered instead of oral acyclovir. Acyclovir ointment, however, may decrease visual acuity and does not prevent viral replication in trigeminal ganglia. For these reasons, the majority of ophthalmologist prescribe oral antivirals for HSV anterior uveitis cases [23].

6.2 Corticosteroids

Topical corticosteroids control anterior chamber inflammation and also acutely reduce intraocular pressure due to the control of inflammation in the trabecular meshwork. A typical treatment regimen is topical prednisolone acetate 1%, four to eight times a day. Systemic corticosteroids are administered in cases with HSV anterior uveitis and concomitant epithelial keratitis; topical corticosteroids are started after dendritic keratitis heals. Corticosteroids should be tapered off slowly after the control of inflammation because rapid withdrawal of the medication may result in a rebound effect. A low dose of topical corticosteroids should be used indefinitely in some patients to maintain long-term control of their inflammation [23].

6.3 Other medications

A topical cycloplegic agent is typically required to avoid posterior synechiae formation and diminish ocular pain and photophobia. Topical and oral anti-glaucoma agents are often required to control high intraocular pressure, especially during the acute phase of the disease. These ocular antihypertensive medications include topical alpha-adrenergic agonists, topical beta-blockers, and topical or oral carbonic anhydrase inhibitors. Latanoprost should probably be avoided as this drug may potentiate HSV reactivation [23].

7. Long-term outcomes

The visual prognosis of HSV anterior uveitis is favorable when diagnosed promptly and if managed correctly. When the infection involves other ocular structures, however, the potential for profound visual loss is enormous. The most serious visual complications of HSV include neurotrophic keratitis, progressive outer retinal necrosis syndrome, and acute retinal necrosis. It is advisable to perform a dilated retinal examination for every case with HSV anterior uveitis to exclude any posterior segment involvement. Long-term use of topical corticosteroids may result in serious complications, including cataracts and glaucoma [4].

8. Future direction

New methods of HSV detection have been introduced recently. Specific circulating microRNAs (miRNAs) can be identified for herpesviruses, without a need for invasive intraocular sampling [24]. In addition, miRNA expression profiles are capable of differentiating latent infection from the active stage of the disease [25]. Artificial intelligence can be part of the future of uveitis diagnosis and management; through combining all data, including clinical signs, ocular imaging, circulating miRNA, and molecular analysis of aqueous humor, machine learning can play an important role in the diagnosis and management algorithms of HSV uveitis.

Novel treatment strategies should target key parameters within the inflammatory pathway that control the initiation and resolution phase of HSV infection. The current therapeutic agents cannot eradicate HSV when it establishes a ganglionic latency in the trigeminal nerve. In theory, immunization against the virus should reduce the incidence of HSV-related eye diseases. Although several candidate HSV vaccines have been tested in humans, currently there are no licensed vaccines against either HSV type.

Treatment for HSV anterior uveitis often requires systemic antiviral agents despite being confined to the eye. This results in issues regarding compliance and systemic adverse reactions, especially in a group of cases that need maintenance treatment to prevent disease recurrence. Local drug delivery systems may be a complementing method to enhance patients' compliance, safety profiles, and cost-effectiveness. Two important issues should be addressed in local therapeutics development, including new delivery systems for the release of drugs in the form of a slow-release insert and drug formulation that enables anti-viral activity without inducing ocular side effects.

9. Conclusion

HSV anterior uveitis usually occurs as a result of recurrent infection rather than primary infection. Viral replication and T cell-mediated response both play a role in the pathogenesis of HSV anterior uveitis, which is an acute, recurrent, and typically unilateral ocular inflammation. Each episode of recurrence is associated with blurred vision, ocular pain, photophobia, and redness. In the absence of active keratitis, the diagnosis of HSV anterior uveitis is based on clinical features, including recurrent episodes of inflammation in the same eye, high intraocular pressure during the inflammatory attacks, localized or diffuse granulomatous KPs, and patchy or sectoral iris atrophy. Confirmation of the diagnosis relies on molecular analyses of aqueous humor, but characteristic clinical findings and high index of suspicion are crucial for early diagnosis and management in routine practice. Oral antivirals and topical corticosteroids have become the main standards for treatment. The visual prognosis of HSV anterior uveitis is favorable when diagnosed promptly and if managed correctly. Long-term oral acyclovir treatment and close follow-up are essential to reduce the burden of the disease and its complications.

Conflict of interest

The authors declare no conflict of interest.

Author details

Sepehr Feizi*, Sahba Fekri and Kiana Hassanpour
Ocular Tissue Engineering Research Center, Research Institute for Ophthalmology and Vision Science, Shahid Beheshti University of Medical Sciences, Tehran, Iran

*Address all correspondence to: sepehrfeizi@yahoo.com

References

[1] Rathinam SR. Global variation and pattern changes in epidemiology of uveitis cases. Indian Journal of Ophthalmology. 2007;**55**:173-183

[2] De-la-Torre A, Valdes-Camacho J, Foster CS. Bilateral herpes simplex uveitis: Review of the literature an own reports. Ocular Immunology and Inflammation. 2016;**25**:1-6

[3] Wensing B, Mochizuki M, De Boer JH. Clinical characteristics of herpes simplex virus associated anterior uveitis. Ocular Immunology and Inflammation. 2018;**26**(3):333-337

[4] Wensing B, Relvas LM, Caspers LE, et al. Comparison of rubella virus- and herpes virus-associated anterior uveitis: Clinical manifestations and visual prognosis. Ophthalmology. 2011;**118**(10):1905-1910

[5] Takase H, Kubono R, Terada Y, et al. Comparison of the ocular characteristics of anterior uveitis caused by herpes simplex, varicella-zoster virus, and cytomegalovirus. Japanese Journal of Ophthalmology. 2014;**58**:473-482

[6] Neumann R, Barequet D, Rosenblatt A, et al. Herpetic anterior uveitis - analysis of presumed and PCR proven cases. Ocular Immunology and Inflammation. 2019;**27**(2):211-218

[7] De Groot-Mijnes JDF, Chan ASY, Chee SP, et al. Immunopathology of virus-induced anterior uveitis. Ocular Immunology and Inflammation. 2018;**26**(3):338-346

[8] Pleyer U, Chee SP. Current aspects on the management of viral uveitis in immunocompetent individuals. Clinical Ophthalmology. 2015;**9**:1017-1028

[9] Jap A, Chee SP. Viral anterior uveitis. Current Opinion in Ophthalmology. 2011;**22**:483-488

[10] Ouwendijk WJ, Laing KJ, Verjans GM, et al. T-cell immunity to human alphaherpesviruses. Current Opinion in Virology. 2013;**3**:452-460

[11] Lee S, Ives AM, Bertke AS. Herpes simplex virus 1 reactivates from autonomic ciliary ganglia independently from sensory trigeminal ganglia to cause recurrent ocular disease. Journal of Virology. 2015;**89**:8383-8391

[12] Richter ER, Dias JK, Gilbert JE 2nd, Atherton SS. Distribution of herpes simplex virus type 1 and varicella zoster virus in ganglia of the human head and neck. The Journal of Infectious Diseases. 2009;**200**:1901-1906

[13] Takase H, Futagami Y, Yoshida T, et al. Cytokine profile in aqueous humor and sera of patients with infectious or noninfectious uveitis. Investigative Ophthalmology & Visual Science. 2006;**47**:1557-1561

[14] Van Der Lelij A, Ooijman FM, Kijlstra A, et al. Anterior uveitis with sectoral iris atrophy in the absence of keratitis: A distinct clinical entity among herpetic eye diseases. Ophthalmology. 2000;**107**(6):1164-1170

[15] Miserocchi E, Fogliato G, Bianchi I, et al. Clinical features of ocular herpetic infection in an Italian referral center. Cornea. 2014;**33**(6):565-570

[16] Choi JA, Ju HH, Kim JE, et al. Cytokine profile and cytoskeletal changes after herpes simplex virus type 1 infection in human trabecular meshwork cells. Journal of Cellular and Molecular Medicine. 2021;**25**(19):9295-9305

[17] Pohlmann D, Pahlitzsch M, Schlickeiser S, et al. Virus-associated anterior uveitis and secondary glaucoma: Diagnostics, clinical characteristics, and surgical options. PLoS One. 2020;**15**(2):e0229260. DOI: 10.1371/journal.pone.0229260 eCollection 2020

[18] Accorinti M, Petitti L, Gaeta A, et al. Viral acute anterior uveitis: clinical signs useful for differential diagnosis. Ocular Immunology and Inflammation. 2021;**29**(7-8):1355-1362

[19] van Boxtel LAA, van der Lelij A, van der Meer J, et al. Cytomegalovirus as a cause of anterior uveitis in immunocompetent patients. Ophthalmology. 2007;**114**(7):1358-1362

[20] Tombolini B, Menean M, Cicinelli MV, et al. Diagnostic and therapeutic results of aqueous real-time polymerase chain reaction in infectious uveitis. Canadian Journal of Ophthalmology. Jun 12, 2023. S0008-4182(23)00173-4. DOI: 10.1016/j.jcjo.2023.05.011. Online ahead of print

[21] Jdf DG-M, Rothova A, Van Loon AM, et al. Polymerase chain reaction and Goldmann-Witmer coefficient analysis are complimentary for the diagnosis of infectious uveitis. American Journal of Ophthalmology. 2006;**141**:313-318

[22] Sugita S, Shimizu N, Watanabe K, et al. Use of multiplex PCR and real-time PCR to detect human herpes virus genome in ocular fluids of patients with uveitis. The British Journal of Ophthalmology. 2008;**92**:928-932

[23] Testi I, Aggarwal K, Jaiswal N, et al. Antiviral therapy for varicella zoster virus (VZV) and herpes simplex virus (HSV)-induced anterior uveitis: A systematic review and meta-analysis. Frontiers in Medicine (Lausanne). 2021;**8**:686427. DOI: 10.3389/fmed.2021.686427

[24] Verma P, Pandey RK, Prajapati P, et al. Circulating MicroRNAs: Potential and emerging biomarkers for diagnosis of human infectious diseases. Frontiers in Microbiology. 2016;**7**:1274

[25] Tribolet L, Kerr E, Cowled C, et al. MicroRNA biomarkers for infectious diseases: From basic research to biosensing. Frontiers in Microbiology. 2020;**11**:1197

Chapter 3

Juvenile Idiopathic Arthritis-Associated Uveitis: Evidence-Based Screening, Monitoring, and Treatment

Luiza M. Neves and Marcela Bohn de A. Alves

Abstract

Juvenile idiopathic arthritis (JIA) is the most frequent chronic autoimmune rheumatic disease in children and adolescents. JIA-associated uveitis is its commonest extra-articular manifestation comprising usually a silent iridocyclitis. Due to this asymptomatic clinical presentation, it is estimated that one-third of JIA-associated uveitis may present with ocular complications by the time of diagnosis. Time-appropriate screening and monitoring are crucial for the prevention of sight-threatening ocular manifestations. Updated treatment is also essential for adequate management and, therefore, to guarantee the best long-term functional vision in these patients. The scope of this chapter involves: (a) JIA and JIA-uveitis introduction/background; (b) etiology, pathogenesis, and risk factors; (c) diagnosis, clinical presentation, and ocular complications; (d) monitoring and screening (including national/international screening guidelines); (e) management (treatment options and treatment monitoring); (f) disease burden; and (g) conclusion and take-home messages.

Keywords: juvenile idiopathic arthritis, anterior uveitis, pediatric uveitis, chronic anterior uveitis, childhood

1. Introduction

Juvenile idiopathic arthritis (JIA) is the most common rheumatic disease in children and adolescents. It comprehends a heterogeneous group of autoimmune arthritis with onset before 16 years of age and a duration of at least 6 weeks (**Table 1**) [1].

Uveitis is the most frequent extra-articular manifestation of JIA, affecting up to one-third of patients within 7 years of the onset of arthritis, although the prevalence of uveitis can vary according to the disease group, being as high as 57% in the young oligoarticular onset subpopulation [2, 3]. JIA-associated uveitis is also the most common cause of uveitis in the pediatric population, representing around 20% of the cases [4, 5].

JIA category	Definition		Prevalence		
			ACR	EULAR	ILAR
Oligoarthritis	Arthritis with 1–4 joints during the first 6 months of disease	Persistent: 1–4 joints	15.6%	17.6%	16.4%
		Extended: >4 joints after the first 6 months of disease			
Polyarthritis	Arthritis with >4 joints during the first 6 months of disease	RF negative	6.2%	8.1%	4.2%
		RF positive on at least two occasions more than 3 months apart	1.9%	1.7%	0.6%
Psoriatic arthritis	Arthritis and psoriasis or arthritis and at least two of: dactylitis; nail pitting or onycholysis; psoriasis in a first-degree relative		4.1%	1.1%	1.1%
Enthesitis-related arthritis	Arthritis and enthesitis or arthritis or enthesitis with at least two of: presence or a history of sacroiliac joint tenderness and/or inflammatory lumbosacral pain; presence of HLA-B27 onset of arthritis in a male older than 6 years of age; acute symptomatic anterior uveitis; history of ankylosing spondylitis, enthesitis-related arthritis, sacroiliitis with inflammatory bowel disease, Reiter's syndrome or acute anterior uveitis in a first-degree relative		13.8%	1.5%	3.1%
Systemic	Arthritis with or preceded by daily fever of at least 2 weeks' duration that is documented to be quotidian for at least 3 days and accompanied by one or more of: evanescent nonfixed erythematous rash; generalized lymph node enlargement; hepatomegaly and/or splenomegaly; serositis		6.4%	2.7%	2.4%
Undifferentiated	Arthritis that fulfills criteria in no category or in two or more of the above categories				2.7%

ACR: American College for Rheumatology; EULAR: European League Against Rheumatism; ILAR: International League of Associations for Rheumatology.

Table 1.
Table extracted from Neves et al. [6] with definitions of JIA categories and prevalence of uveitis for each JIA category defined by ACR, EULAR, and ILAR classification [7, 8].

JIA-associated uveitis more commonly manifests itself presents as an asymptomatic chronic anterior uveitis without external evidence of inflammation, and a delayed diagnosis can result in sight-threatening complications, which can be seen in one-third of cases at presentation, and up to 67% of cases over all [9]. Ocular complications include band keratopathy, anterior and posterior synechia, glaucoma, cataract and macular edema, and scaring.

Differently, specific HLA B27-associated uveitis in children with spondyloarthritis typically presents as a symptomatic acute anterior uveitis which is often episodic and does not require systemic treatment [10].

The visual prognosis of children with JIA-associated uveitis can be very poor, with reports of severe sight loss and sight impairment varying from 9 to 22% [2, 11]. Early detection and appropriate treatment of uveitis are of utmost importance to avoid the development of sight-threatening irreversible complications and prevent permanent visual loss. International guidelines for JIA-affected children and young people have been developed as an attempt to reduce this burden.

In this chapter, we aim to revise this important cause of uveitis in the pediatric population, its clinical presentation, management, and the disease burden associated with it.

2. Epidemiology, pathogenesis, and risk-factors

2.1 Epidemiology

JIA incidence varies from 1.6 to 23/100,000 and JIA prevalence varies from 3.8 to 400/100,000 [8]. Oligoarthritis is its most frequent form. The pooled incidence and prevalence are higher for girls (10.0 [9.4–10.7]/100,000 and 19.4 [18.3–20.6]/100,000) than for boys (5.7 [5.3–6.2]/100,000 and 11.0 [10.2–11.9]/100,000) [8]. JIA-associated uveitis incidence is estimated in 1/100.000 [12].

The effect of ethnicity is unclear and JIA-associated uveitis seems to be more frequent in Caucasians than in Afro-American children and adolescents. Also, geographical differences show a higher JIA prevalence in Europe and North America than in Asia [7]. Nevertheless, this should be interpreted with caution as there is scarce epidemiological data in other areas such as Latin America and Africa.

2.2 Pathogenesis

The pathogenesis of JIA-uveitis is still not fully understood. What is currently known is its multifactorial immune-mediated background with complex genetic and environmental factors involving concealed infection, psychological stress, vitamin D deficiency, or use of specific vaccines [13].

Histocompatibility allele profiles have been widely assessed and human leukocyte antigen (HLA)-DRB*03, *08, *11, *12, *13, and *14 were associated with an increased risk of uveitis in JIA patients [13]. By contrast, the HLA-DR1 haplotype and HLA-DQA*0101 allele seem to be protective. HLA-B27, which is associated with enthesitis-related arthritis, confers an increased risk of acute anterior uveitis (AAU) [14].

Regarding genetic traits, there have been few reports of familial cases of JIA-uveitis, as there is a lack of a single-gene, mendelian trait of inheritance, suggesting also a complex genetic pathogenesis [15].

Interestingly, children with JIA-uveitis revealed higher levels of cytokines and chemokines (IL-2, IL-6, IL-13, IL-18, IFN-γ, TNF, soluble ICAM-1 (also known as CD54), C-C motif chemokine 5 (CCL5, also known as RANTES) and C-X-C motif chemokine 10 (CXCL10, also known as IP-10) in the aqueous humor than ones without uveitis [16].

2.3 Risk factors

It is well established that JIA-uveitis has several risk factors which are: age at arthritis onset, gender, JIA subtype, antinuclear antibody (ANA) positivity, human leukocytes antigen (HLA)-B27 positivity, and anti-histone antibodies (AHA) 15 U/mL [1, 9, 17].

These risk factors are different depending on the course (acute or chronic) of the uveitis. Chronic anterior uveitis (CAU) is associated with less than 6 years old at JIA onset, female gender, oligoarticular disease (four or fewer joints at disease onset), and ANA positivity, which occurs in 70–90% of JIA-uveitis cases [1, 9]. However, it seems that age-dependent risk of developing uveitis is related only for girls and not for boys [17, 18].

In contrast, AAU is associated with pre-teenaged and teenaged patients, male gender, enthesitis-related arthritis, and positive HLA-B27 [1, 7]. Uveitis can also be observed in patients with rheumatoid factor (RF)-negative polyarthritis, psoriatic arthritis, and, more rarely, in systemic-onset JIA [7]. In this regard, the polyarticular RF positivity subtype was revealed as protective for uveitis [9].

JIA-associated uveitis with risk of poor prognosis is associated with specific risk factors that should be mentioned, such as male sex, younger age at JIA-uveitis onset, short duration between onset of arthritis and uveitis (median 6 months), development of uveitis prior to arthritis, presence of synechiae, high anterior chamber cell grade (>2+), and poor visual acuity at uveitis diagnosis [19].

3. Diagnosis, clinical presentation, and ocular complications

Uveitis is the presenting complaint in 3–7% of patients with JIA, whereas in most cases arthritis precedes the uveitis by a mean of 4–5 months. Most patients that develop uveitis (73%) will do so in the first year after their arthritis diagnosis [20].

The most common manifestation of JIA-uveitis is as an asymptomatic, bilateral, non-granulomatous iridocyclitis [21]. Usually, its onset is insidious, its duration is persistent (lasts more than 3 months) and its course is chronic (relapse in less than 3 after discontinuing treatment) in up to 90% of cases [21]. In contrast, some subgroups can present with AAU (10–16.2% of cases), as those associated with HLA B27-related enthesitis. Panuveitis has rarely been described [21].

The diagnosis of JIA-uveitis is performed clinically during an ophthalmological examination mostly done at the slit-lamp, with the identification of signs of anterior chamber inflammation (cells and/or flare) or its complications. Smaller or uncooperative children may require the use of portable slit lamps or indirect ophthalmoscope for assessment.

As the CAU is typically asymptomatic with no external evidence of inflammation, one-third of patients will have ocular complications on diagnosis, and up to 67% of them will develop complication during the course of their disease [9]. Poor prognosis factors include severe disease at presentation, uveitis preceding arthritis and male gender [22, 23]. Anterior chamber flare is also considered an important marker of disease gravity in children, and its presence can be predictive of adverse events during the disease's course [24].

Additionally, the fact that most children and young people will not notice changes in vision or symptoms until complications are present can lead to difficult treatment adhesion, especially in cases where the severity of the uveitis is more significant than the arthritis and guides their treatment.

3.1 Posterior synechiae

Posterior synechiae are adherences between the iris and lens which occur due to fibrin exudation in significant anterior chamber inflammatory processes [25]. They are a common complication (27–33%) that can collaborate with the increased intraocular pressure and accelerate cataract formation (see below) and have been independently associated with decreased vision [26].

3.2 Band keratopathy

Chronic degenerative condition is frequently associated with chronic ocular inflammation; it is characterized by the deposition of calcium in hydroxyapatite form into superficial layers of the cornea and is present in 15–29% of patients. These grayish-to-whitish opacities first appear peripherally in the corneal surface (3 h and 9 h), extending centrally to form coalescent dense plaques in the interpalpebral zone, affecting the visual axis and causing ocular discomfort (**Figure 1**) [27].

3.3 Cataract

Cataract formation is the most common ocular complication associated with visual impairment and occurs in about a third of the cases [25]. It is a consequence of chronic inflammation and topical and systemic corticosteroid use. The risk of cataract development with topical steroid use seems to be independent of the presence of active uveitis and posterior synechiae, and it increases as more drops are used over longer periods of time (especially if >3 drops daily) [28, 29].

Particular attention must be given to pre-school children with asymmetrical cataracts due to the risk of amblyopia.

3.4 Glaucoma or ocular hypertension

Ocular hypertension is defined as intra-ocular pressure of more than 21 mmHg in three consecutive measurements, or a single measurement of 30 mmHg or more [30]. It can be a result of a dysfunctional trabecular meshwork due to chronic anterior uveitis, a steroid response to topical (mainly) or systemic treatment with corticosteroids, or a combination of all. Its prevalence varies from 8 to 19% in JIA-associated uveitis. The presence of synechiae and pupillary seclusion can also compromise the aqueous humor outflow and collaborate to that. The use of 0.1% dexamethasone eye drops four times a day for more than 8 weeks can result in ocular

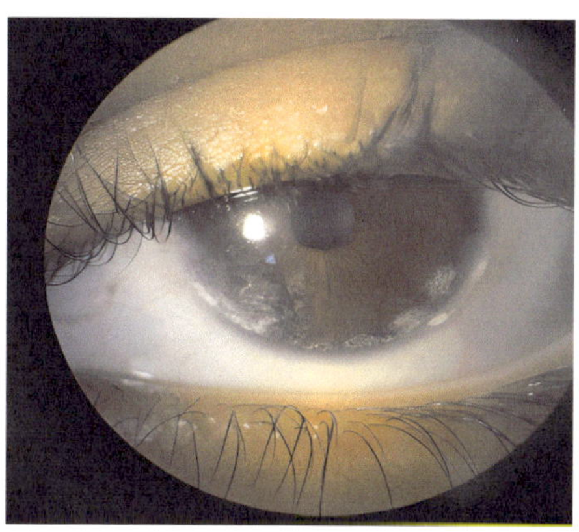

Figure 1.
Peripheral band keratopathy.

hypertension in 60–70% of patients [29]. Secondary glaucoma occurs when there is optic glaucomatous nerve damage and visual field defects as a consequence of ocular hypertension.

3.5 Hypotony

Hypotony is defined by an intraocular pressure of less than 5 mmHg and results from severe ciliary body inflammation and/or atrophy. Although not as common as the previous complications (7.1–9.3%), it is associated with more severe uveitic disease, panuveitis, and the presence of posterior synechiae, and can lead to poor visual outcomes due to hypotony maculopathy and papillopathy and end-stage shrinking of the eye (phthisis bulbi) [31]. Early start of immunosupressive therapy seems to have a protective effect against the development of hypotony [31].

3.6 Macular edema

Macular edema is defined as an increase in central macular thickness, and can be related to inflammatory stress, microvascular changes, be a complication of cataract, other intra-ocular surgeries, or hypotony (**Figure 2**). Its prevalence is estimated in 6–25% of cases [32]. The duration of JIA-uveitis positively correlates with the development of macular edema [32]. The widespread use of optical coherence tomography (OCT) as part of the routine ocular exam has led to early detection of macular thickness changes, facilitating disease activity monitoring.

3.7 Papillitis

Often seen as a sign of inflammatory activity rather than a complication, it is often present in cases of severe anterior uveitis in children (12%), and is not necessarily

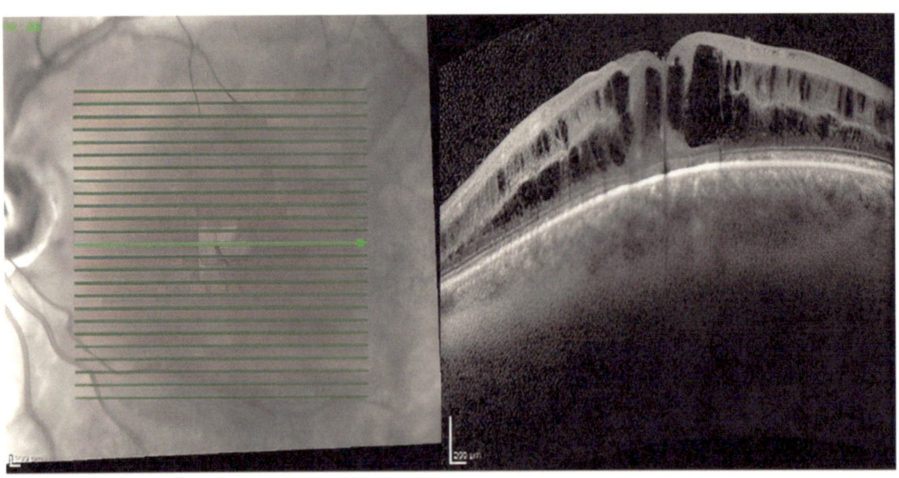

Figure 2.
Left chronic macular edema at OCT.

associated with primarily intermediate or posterior uveitis, as in adults. It seems to be more present in boys than girls, and not independently related to worse visual acuity [33]. Clinically, optic nerve function tends to be preserved, with normal color vision and no red desaturation, and optic nerve imaging such as retinal nerve fiber layer thickness on OCT can be a useful monitoring tool.

4. Screening and monitoring

4.1 Screening

Ophthalmological screening is recommended when JIA is suspected or within the first 6 weeks of final diagnosis [34, 35] or, if symptomatic, within 1 week of referral [35]. Current literature has different recommendations regarding the frequency of ophthalmological screening after this first examination and they can be seen in **Table 2**.

Based on the British Society for Pediatric and Adolescent Rheumatology/Royal College of Ophthalmology (BSPAR/RCO) guidelines, the ophthalmological screening of uveitis frequency should be every 2 months for 6 months followed by every 3–4 months [35]. The duration of these examinations will be determined according to the patient's age and to the type of JIA, as is described in **Table 2**.

Based on the American College of Rheumatology/Arthritis Foundation (ACR/AF) guidelines and also on the Brazilian Society of Pediatric Ophthalmology (SBOP) recommendations (**Table 2** and **Figure 3**), patients with JIA are classified as high, moderate, and low risk for developing uveitis [36]. High-risk patients include those with oligoarthritis, polyarthritis with negative RF, psoriatic arthritis, and undifferentiated arthritis, those with positive ANA, younger than 7 years of age at JIA onset, and with a disease duration of less than 4 years [36]. Low to moderate-risk patients are those with JIA in the aforementioned categories but with negative ANA, older than 7 years at JIA onset or with more than 4 years of disease duration, and those with systemic JIA, positive RF-polyarthritis, and enthesitis-related arthritis [6, 36]. Based on this, high-risk uveitis patients should be screened every 3 months and low- to moderate-risk uveitis patients every 6–12 months (**Table 2** and **Figure 3**) [36]. Follow-up should be until 11 years old or according to medical criteria [6].

According to the Brazilian Medical Association (AMB) and the Brazilian Society of Rheumatology (SBR) guidelines, ocular screening should start at the time of JIA diagnosis [37]. Its frequency should be based on JIA subtype, age at the disease onset, disease duration, and positive ANA, as shown in **Table 2**.

Ophthalmological screening exams should include age-appropriate visual acuity tests, classification of the anterior chamber cell grade inflammation at the slit lamp by the Standardization of Uveitis Nomenclature Working Group (SUN) criteria and quantification of structural complications [38]. In addition, recording the duration of active inflammation and detailing the treatment response are also important for JIA-uveitis monitoring [39].

4.2 Monitoring

Therefore, ophthalmological screening is indicated in JIA patients without uveitis. For children and adolescents with uveitis-JIA, it is important to differentiate, at the examination, if the uveitis is controlled or uncontrolled.

	BSPAR/RCO	ACR/AF/SBOP			BSRP
First exam	Before 6 weeks of diagnosis; If symptomatic: within a week of referral	No recommendations (ACR/AF) When JIA is suspected or diagnosis within 6 weeks of diagnosis			At JIA diagnosis
Freq.	Every 2 m for 6 m Followed by every 3–4 m for (see below):	Oligoarthritis, polyarthritis and negative RF, psoriatic arthritis and undifferentiated arthritis		Systemic JIA, polyarthritis and positive RF Enthesitis-related arthritis	JIA age of onset ≤6 y, disease duration ≤4 y, oligo/poly and ANA positive Every 3 m.
	Oligoarticular JIA, psoriatic arthritis and enthesitis-related arthritis despite ANA status onset under 11 y: < 3 y onset: 8 y 3–4 y onset: 6 y 5–8 y onset: 3 y 9–10 y onset: 1y	PositiveANA, JIA age of onset <7 y and disease duration ≤4 y	NegativeANA, JIA age onset ≥7 y or disease duration >4 y		JIA age of onset ≤6 y, disease duration ≤4 y. Oligo/poly, negative ANA or JIA age of onset ≤6 y disease duration >4 y, oligo/polyarthritis, despite ANA status or JIA age of onset >6 y, disease duration ≤4 y, oligo/poly, despite ANA status Every 6 m
	Polyarticular, positive ANA, JIA onset less than 10 y < 6 y onset: 5 y 6–9 y onset: 2 y				
	Polyarticular, positive ANA JIA, JIA onset less than 7 y: 5 y	Every 3 m	Every 6–12 m		Systemic JIA, polyarthritis with positive RF, and enthesitis-related arthritis or JIA age of onset ≤6 y, duration of JIA ≥ 7 y oligo/polyarthritis, despite ANA status or JIA age of onset >6 y, duration of JIA > 4 y, oligo/polyarthritis, despite ANA status Every 12 m.

Freq.: frequency; JIA: juvenile idiopathic arthritis; m: months; y: years; ANA: antinuclear antibody; RF: rheumatoid factor.

Table 2.
Table extracted from Neves et al. [6] Screening criteria for ophthalmological examination in juvenile idiopathic arthritis by the British Society for Pediatric and Adolescent Rheumatology/Royal College of Ophthalmology (BSPAR/RCO), the American College of Rheumatology/Arthritis Foundation (ACR/AF), the Brazilian Society of Pediatric Ophthalmology (SBOP), and the Brazilian Society of Rheumatologic Pediatrician (BSRP) Guideline and [6, 35–37].

Uncontrolled uveitis occurs when there is an increase of anterior chamber cells to grade 1+ or more, or new signs of inflammation/complications of inflammation [36]. Controlled uveitis is considered when there are no or grade < 1+ anterior chamber cells without new complications due to active inflammation; absence of optic disc, macular edema, and vitreous haze [36].

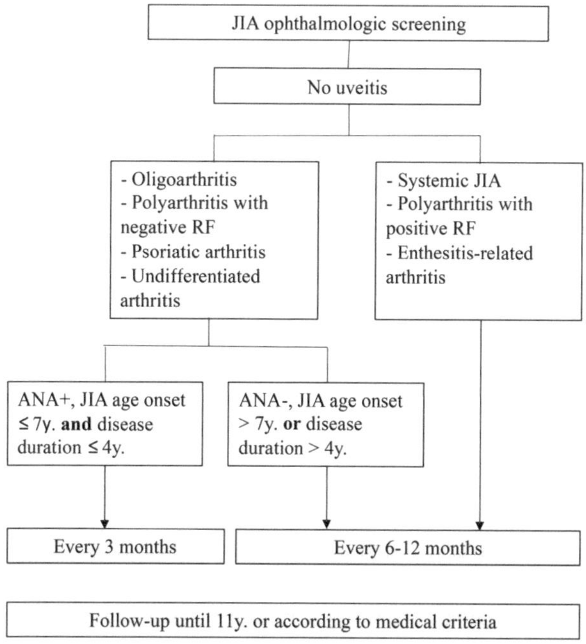

Figure 3.
Figure extracted from Neves et al. [6]: Ophthalmological screening in juvenile idiopathic arthritis.

The frequency of ophthalmological monitoring in uncontrolled uveitis should be according to the anterior chamber degree of inflammation classification by SUN (**Figure 4**) [36, 40]:

In grades 3+ or 4+: weekly until improvement.

In grades 1+ or 2+ (stable in two successive visits): every 2 weeks (or at least in less than 6 weeks).

In grade 0.5+ (stable in two successive visits): every 6 weeks (or at least in less than 3 months).

Naturally, this follow-up frequency is a suggestion and ophthalmological monitoring in uncontrolled uveitis should also be individualized based on clinical factors such as the frequency of topical glucocorticoid administration, the IOP, and the presence of ocular complications [36].

The recommendations for ophthalmological monitoring in children and adolescents with controlled JIA-uveitis can be divided into who is tapering/discontinuing therapy (topical or systemic) and who has stable therapy (**Figure 4**) [36]:

Tapering or discontinuing topical glucocorticoids: monitoring should be monthly. Also, the patient should be evaluated before each step of tapering.

Tapering or discontinuing systemic therapy: within 2 months. In the suspension of systemic or immunomodulatory therapy, monitoring should be performed every 2 months for 6 months.

Stable therapy, systemic or topical: every 3 months.

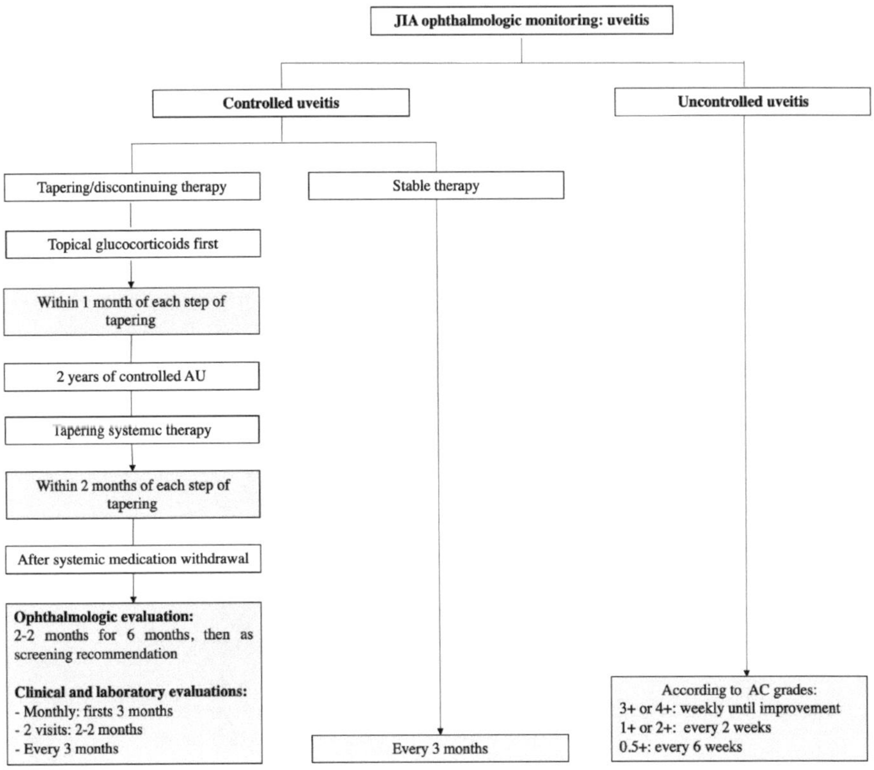

Figure 4.
Figure extracted from Neves et al. [6]: Ophthalmological monitoring in juvenile idiopathic arthritis-related uveitis.

5. Management (treatment options and monitoring)

5.1 Topical therapy

Topical glucocorticoids are the first-line treatment for JIA-uveitis, acute or chronic uveitis. Prednisolone acetate 1% eye drop is the topical glucocorticoid of choice due to its good corneal penetration and low risk of IOP elevation (**Figure 5**) [1, 36]. The frequency of the administration is based on the degree of anterior chamber inflammation. Topical and systemic nonsteroidal anti-inflammatory therapy should not be used as single therapy [41].

The cycloplegic eye drop, tropicamide 10 mg/ml, should also be given to prevent or treat posterior synechiae in active uveitis in a recommended frequency of one drop every 8 hours. Its adverse events include somnolence, reduced accommodation, and blurred vision.

Topical treatment should be maintained as long as there are ≥0.5+ cells in the anterior chamber. However, prolonged topical glucocorticoids therapy has potential ocular adverse effects. Therefore, in patients who are not on systemic therapy, but still require one to two drops of topical glucocorticoids daily for uveitis control over 3 months, it is recommended to add systemic therapy, described in the next item [1, 36] Eventually, in the absence of ocular complications, such as elevated IOP and cataract, and guaranteeing regular ocular follow-up, topical glucocorticoids at a dosage of one to two drops daily may be used as monotherapy [36].

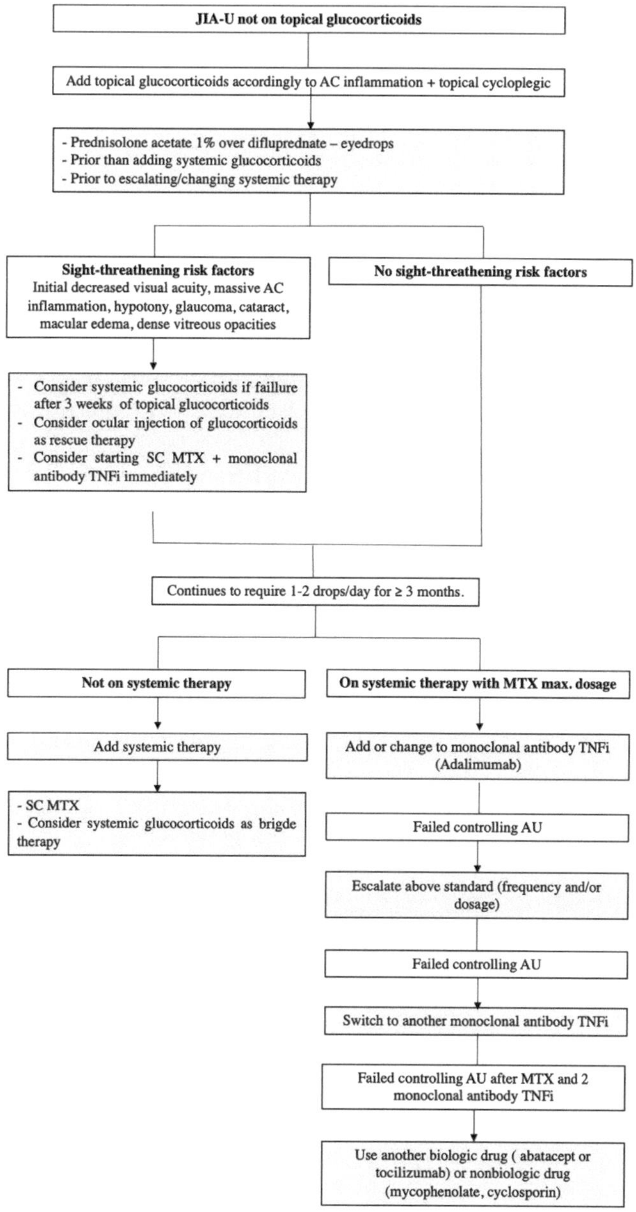

Figure 5.
Figure extracted from Neves et al. [6]: Treatment steps in juvenile idiopathic arthritis-related uveitis.

Subtenon or orbital floor injection of glucocorticoids as a rescue therapy has been suggested in selected cases such as in unilateral or bilateral severe (3+ or 4+ AC cells) or refractory (after 2 weeks of topical and oral corticosteroids without clinical improvement) uveitis, especially in patients with sight-threatening risk factors [40, 41]. These risk factors include initial decreased visual acuity, massive anterior chamber inflammation, hypotony, glaucoma, cataract, dense vitreous opacities, or macular edema.

The injection dosage is 2–4 mg of dexamethasone phosphate or 20–40 mg of triamcinolone acetonide. The intravitreal injection dosage is 700 mg of a dexamethasone phosphate implant and 2–4 mg of triamcinolone acetonide. However, intraocular glucocorticoids are associated with cataract development and a risk of increased IOP, and IOP should be monitored weekly [40, 41].

5.2 Systemic therapy

Systemic treatment is usually indicated in JIA-uveitis in two scenarios: (a) when there is a failure of adequate control of inflammation after 3 months of topical treatment [1, 36] and (b) after 3 weeks without uveitis control in the presence of sight-threatening risk factors such as initial decreased visual acuity, massive anterior chamber inflammation, hypotony, glaucoma, cataract, dense vitreous opacities, or macular edema [40].

Systemic treatment options include glucocorticoid, disease-modifying anti-rheumatic drugs (DMARDs) (methotrexate, mycophenolate mofetil, cyclosporine A, and azathioprine), and biological agents (anti-tumor necrosis factor [anti-TNF] blockers: adalimumab, infliximab, golimumab, etanercept; CTLA4-Ig: abatacept; and anti-IL6: tocilizumab) (**Table 3**).

Drug name	Mechanism	Preferred dosage and route	Ocular and systemic side effects	Laboratory routine
Synthetic DMARDs				
Methotrexate	Cellular adenosine release	10–15 mg/m^2 BS PO or SC weekly. Adjust dose gradually to achieve an optimal response.	GI discomfort, nausea, diarrhea, photosensitivity, rash, increased AST or ALT, cytopenias.	Baseline: Complete blood and platelet count Renal function Liver function Chest X-ray Monitoring: Hemogram, renal and liver function tests every 1–3 month.
Mycophenolate mofetil	Inhibitor of inosine-5-monophosphate dehydrogenase	300 mg/m^2 bd, increasing to 600 mg/m^2 bd	GI discomfort, leukopenia, pure red cell aplasia, hair loss, lymphoma and malignancy (particularly of the skin)	Complete blood cell counts weekly during the first month, twice monthly for the second and third months and then monthly
Cyclosporine A	Calcineurin inhibitor blocking T-cell proliferation	2.5–5 mg/kg/day in 2 doses	GI disturbance, hypertension, renal and liver dysfunctions, lipid abnormalities, hirsutism, gum hypertrophy	Renal and liver functions, serum lipids, magnesium and potassium. Cyclosporine blood concentration adjusted to 100 mcg/dl
Azathioprine	Purine nucleoside analogue, inhibits DNA replication	1–3 mg/kg/day	Myelotoxicity and hepatotoxicity.	Complete blood and platelet count, liver function tests every 1–3 months

Drug name	Mechanism	Preferred dosage and route	Ocular and systemic side effects	Laboratory routine
Biological DMARDs				
Adalimumab	Anti-TNF alfa/ human monoclonal antibody	Body weight 10–15 kg: 10 mg SC every other week 15–30 kg: 20 mg SC every other week ≥30 kg: 40 mg SC every other week	Opportunistic infections by *Legionella*, *Listeria*, tuberculosis, and invasive fungal infections. Hepatitis B virus reactivation. Infusion reaction. Hepatotoxicity (infliximab and tocilizumab). Heart failure. Hypersensitivity and anaphylaxis. Risk of cancer (invasive cervical cancer, hepatosplenic T-cell lymphoma). Cytopenias. Lupus-like syndrome. Demyelinating disease. Gastrointestinal perforation (tocilizumab). Vitreous hemorrhage (adalimumab and infliximab)	Check for latent infection. Avoid live vaccines during treatment or offer live vaccines prior to treatment. Complete blood count. Hepatic function (infliximab and tocilizumab).
Infliximab	Anti-TNF alpha/ chimeric (mouse-human monoclonal antibody)	Initially 6 mg/kg/dose IV 3–10 mg/kg/dose IV at 2 weeks, then every 4–8 weeks, adjusted according to response		
Tocilizumab	Anti-IL-6/ humanized monoclonal antibody	Body weight < 30 kg: 10 mg/kg IV[6] body weight > 30 kg: 8 mg/kg IV[6] every 4 weeks		
Abatacept	Inhibition of lymphocyte co-stimulation (CTLA4)/ human fusion protein	10 mg/kg IV At weeks 0, 2, 4, and every 4 weeks		

PO: by mouth; SC: subcutaneous; GI: gastro intestinal; Bd: twice daily; Anti-TNF: anti-tumor necrosis factor; IV: intravenous; IL: interleukin; CTLA4: cytotoxic T-lymphocyte-associated protein 4.

Table 3.
T extracted from Neves et al. [6]: Drug names; mechanism of action; preferred dosage and route; ocular and systemic side effects; adverse events; and laboratory routine of synthetic and biological disease-modifying anti-rheumatic drugs (DMARDs) for juvenile idiopathic arthritis-associated uveitis [1, 41].

Methotrexate (MTX) is the first-line systemic treatment either oral or parenteral (subcutaneous, preferably, or intramuscular routes) [1, 36]. Laboratory routine with transaminases should be performed every 1–3 months. If transaminases increase up to 1 fold the upper limits, MTX dose should be reversed; if transaminases increase more than 2 fold the upper limits, MTX should be suspended for 2–4 weeks and then restarted. Under normal transaminases status, treatment should be resumed otherwise it is recommended its withdrawal (**Table 3**).

Briefly, **Figure 5** summarizes the steps to achieve optimal uveitis control under systemic therapy. Systemic therapy is initiated with MTX. Systemic glucocorticoids may be used as bridge therapy in patients with sight-threatening risk factors until a DAMARD effect can is achieved5 In addition, patients with sight-threatening complications, should initiate treatment with MTX combined with a monoclonal TNF inhibitor [36] (**Table 3**).

If no control of uveitis is observed or the disease worsens after 3–4 months on MTX initial therapy, it is recommended to associate a biological agent [1]. The ACR recommends monoclonal anti-TNF drugs, preferably adalimumab, infliximab, or golimumab [36] (**Table 3**).

If the patient is under one monoclonal anti-TNF at a standard dose and still has active CAU, the recommendation is to escalate the dose and/or frequency to above the standard before switching to another monoclonal anti-TNF [36]. In children and adolescents with active CAU who have failed the first monoclonal anti-TNF with proper dosage and/or frequency, changing to another monoclonal TNF inhibitor is recommended over switching to another biologic category [36] (**Table 3**).

If the patient still has active CAU, despite the use of MTX combined with monoclonal anti-TNF at a higher dosage/frequency, it is recommended to switch to another biological agent of different mechanism of action (abatacept or tocilizumab) or associate with immunomodulatory synthetic agents (mycophenolate, leflunomide, or cyclosporine) [36] (**Table 3**).

Both ophthalmologist and pediatric rheumatologist follow-ups are fundamental for appropriate management of JIA-associated uveitis. Regarding this, vaccination should be completed preferably within 4 weeks before treatment [41]. Tuberculosis and latent tuberculosis infection screening should also be done before initiation of anti-TNF biologics. Drug adherence, contraception for adolescents, and rigorous monitoring for infections and malignancy should also be routinely evaluated [41] (**Table 3**).

Table 3 comprises drug names; mechanism of action; preferred dosage and route; ocular and systemic side effects; adverse events; and laboratory routine of synthetic and biological DMARDs for JIA-associated uveitis [1, 41].

6. Disease burden

JIA and JIA-associated uveitis have a huge impact on the children affected by it. This impact extends not only to the patients, but also to their caregivers and other family members, and imposes a significant burden on different spheres of their lives, even after they reach adulthood. This includes, but is not limited to, their health-related quality of life, physical function, visual outcomes, school attendance, psychological and emotional development as well as the costs involved with long-term treatments and multiple hospital appointments [42]. A study from Germany looked into the direct costs (healthcare and non-healthcare costs) and indirect costs (productivity loss due to sick leave and work disability) for patients with JIA over a 17 year follow-up, and the results showed an estimated mean total cost of €3500 per patient/year [43]. The large majority of the costs (90%) were related to patients with persistently active disease (55%), as well as functional disabilities and certain JIA subgroups, and could reach up to €17,000 a year. Although most healthcare-related costs will vary between countries with different healthcare systems, it is valid to assume that a similar financial burden will fall upon JIA patients worldwide.

Additionally, as these children reach adolescence and young adulthood, the impacts of having a chronic illness and possible disabilities may negatively influence their ability to develop their own identity and independence, as they may need to rely more on their caregivers for financial support and morbidities management than other young people [44].

In patients with JIA, having uveitis has been associated with a worse quality of live. Among JIA-uveitis patients, additional factors that negatively influenced the quality of life were bilateral uveitis, visual impairment and posterior involvement [45]. Other studies looking into the quality of life of pediatric patients with chronic uveitis have shown that the visual loss and fear of blindness are not the only stressors for the patients and their families, as the frequency of eye examinations, treatment regimens and side effects also play an important role. Both the disease and its treatment can interfere with transition to autonomy in adulthood, as reported for other chronic conditions, and problems with treatment adherence are frequent [46]. The development of unified multidisciplinary teams, with joint clinics for all healthcare team involved in their management, seem to have a positive impact on patients and family members [47].

Understanding the impact of the disease and its treatment on a child's or young person's life is of utmost important to allow us to provide better care and support for young patients, and more studies are required to find ways to reduce the disease burden following an hollistic approach [48].

7. Differential diagnosis

Pediatric uveitis represents less than 10% of all uveitis and have a broad etiologic spectrum. It can be classified as idiopathic (majority), infectious (viral, bacterial, parasitic, and less commonly, fungal), non-infectious diseases (mainly autoimmune), and masquerade syndromes (tumoral, non-autoimmune inflammation, retinal dystrophies) [49, 50]. Age, geographic location, and socioeconomic status appear to affect the prevalence of each disease, but it is beyond the scope of this chapter.

It is important to briefly describe the main differential diagnosis of JIA-associated uveitis, as some of the anterior ocular findings may be similar among them. **Table 4** shows the main diseases and their similarities and differences with JIA-uveitis [49, 50].

In the presence of anterior chamber inflammation, it is important to exclude ocular infections such as toxoplasmosis, especially in endemic areas, syphilis, and herpes. Usually, the first two manifest as posterior uveitis with mild to moderate granulomatous anterior uveitis. Herpes simplex infection commonly presents as keratitits or keratouveitis, but more rarely presents as a unilateral painful non-granulomatous anterior uveitis with cornea hypoesthesia, high intra-ocular pressure, and iris atrophy.

Painless CAU can be found not only in JIA, but also in idiopathic causes and familial autosomal dominant hereditary Blau syndrome. In the first case, the anterior uveitis is not associated with any systemic findings, whereas in the second it presents with arthritis, granulomatous ocular signs, chorioretinal lesions, and a family history of similar features, which can mimic ocular sarcoidosis.

Painful AAU is typical of enthesis-related arthritis, sporadic early onset sarcoidosis and tubulointersticial nephritis uveitis syndrome. Each of them has specific systemic findings described in **Table 4**. Less commonly, Behçet disease and Vogt-Koyanagi-Harada syndrome, two causes of panuveitis, should also be remembered as differential diagnosis, although the first one has ocular signs of vasculitis and retinitis and the second one has typical systemic signs of vitiligo, poliosis, dysacusia, as well as typical choroidal involvement.

Less commonly but crucial to point out are the masquerades syndromes, such as retinoblastoma and leukemia, that can manifest as anterior uveitis. Clinical history and complete ophthalmological examination with fundoscopy are essential to their diagnosis.

JIA-uveitis differential diagnosis	Type of uveitis	Systemic findings	Ocular similarities	Ocular differences
Non-infectious uveitis				
Idiopathic anterior uveitis	Anterior uveitis (acute or chronic)	Nothing Exclusion diagnosis	Chronic anterior uveitis	Age of onset 7–12 years, acute anterior uveitis
Enthesis-related arthritis	Acute unilateral anterior uveitis	Enthesitis	Anterior chamber inflammation, complications such as band keratopathy, cataracts, and ocular hypertension	Pain, redness, HLA-B27 positivity
Sporadic early-onset sarcoidosis (onset before age 5)	Acute bilateral anterior uveitis	Multisystemic granulomatous inflammatory disorder. While older children may present with pulmonary involvement, young children typically present with a triad of arthritis, skin (follicular or nodular rash) lesions and uveitis	Anterior chamber inflammation, complications such as band keratopathy (rare), cataracts, and ocular hypertension Lately, chronic anterior uveitis	Pain, anterior chamber granulomatous features (granulomatous keratic precipitates, iris nodules), peripheral and broad-based posterior synechiae, granulomatous optic neuropathy, choroidal involvement (multifocal choroiditis, choroidal granulomas).
Tubulointersticial nephritis uveitis syndrome	Acute bilateral anterior uveitis	Fever, malaise and weight loss. Tubulointerstitial nephritis evidenced by increasing urea and creatinine levels, proteinuria, microhematuria, glycosuria and elevated urinary beta-2-acroglobulin level.	Anterior chamber inflammation	Median age of onset 15 years old, pain, photophobia, there may be anterior chamber granulomatous features, retinal periphlebitis, disc edema, multifocal choroiditis
Pars planitis	Intermediate uveitis	Idiopathic	Mild to moderate anterior segment inflammation, Complications: Band keratopathy, peripheral corneal endotheliopathy, posterior synechiae, less commonly cystoid macular edema.	Age of onset 7–12 years., diffuse vitreous cells and haze, snowballs and snowbanks located inferiorly. Complications such as optic disc edema, neovascularization of the optic disc, inferior peripheral retinoschisis.

JIA-uveitis differential diagnosis	Type of uveitis	Systemic findings	Ocular similarities	Ocular differences
Familial autosomal dominant hereditary Blau Syndrome	Chronic bilateral granulomatous panuveitis with multifocal chorioretinal lesions	Granulomatous polyarthritis + dermatitis+ uveitis; CARD15/NOD2 gene on chromosome 16q12; autosomal dominant pattern	Anterior chamber inflammation and complications	Granulomatous panuveitis with multifocal chorioretinal lesions
Behçet Disease	Panuveitis with retinal vasculitis, retinitis and vascular occlusion.	Recurrent, painful, oropharyngeal and genital ulceration, systemic vasculitis, acne, folliculitis, epididymitis, arthralgia, erythema nodosum, gastrointestinal inflammation.	Mild to moderate non-granulomatous anterior chamber inflammation. Complications such as cataract, intraocular pressure elevation, macular edema or maculopathy, and optic atrophy are the most common complications	Panuveitis with retinal vasculitis and retinitis. Mean onset of 11 years old, HLA B51 positivity
Vogt-Koyanagi-Harada syndrome	Bilateral panuveitis.	Acute meningoencephalitis, vitiligo, poliosis and dysacusia.	Anterior chamber inflammation	Pain, anterior chamber granulomatous features, serous retinal detachment, thick choroids
Infectious uveitis				
Toxoplasmosis	Unifocal and unilateral retinalchoroiditis	Primary infection: mononucleosis-like systemic symptoms	Mild to moderate anterior chamber inflammation	Granulomatous features, retinitis, choriorretinal scar
Syphilis	Usually posterior uveitis but can be anterior, intermediate and panuveitis	Congenital or acquired (sexual abuse)	Mild to moderate anterior chamber inflammation	If congenital, intersticial keratitis. If acquired, diverse presentation
Herpes	Anterior uveitis	Measles-like symptoms	Non-granoloumatous anterior uveitis, although can be granulomatous	Unilateral, pain, dendritic keratitis, cornea hypoesthesia, intersticial keratitis, posterior uveitis with retinitis
Masquerade syndromes				
Retinoblastoma	Leukocoria, strabismus and uveitis	Family history	Anterior uveitis in 0.5–3%	Leukocoria, strabismus, anterior uveitis with pseudohypopyon, neovascular glaucoma, posterior retinal lesions or vitreous seeding

JIA-uveitis differential diagnosis	Type of uveitis	Systemic findings	Ocular similarities	Ocular differences
Leukemia	Anterior or posterior uveitis, chloroma	Weight loss, fever, tiredness, easy bleeding/bruising	Anterior chamber inflammation	Multiple flame retinal hemorrhages (often with white centers) and retinal infiltrates.

Table 4.
JIA-uveitis Differential Diagnosis regarding type of uveitis, systemic findings, ocular similarities and ocular differences.

8. Future directions

Recent efforts have been made to review the currently used JIA classifications to include a more evidence-based approach, that allows the division of the multiple heterogeneous autoimmune arthritis groups in children, into more homogenous clinical groups, based not only on clinical presentation but also routine laboratory tests, and better differentiates these groups from adults presentations [51]. One of the subgroups that require better classification is that of early JIA onset (before 6 years of age) with specific features of female prevalence, symmetric arthritis, anterior uveitis, ANA, and HLA-DR8 positivity. It is expected that a better classification will facilitate research and clinical practice normalization, ultimately allowing for better treatment planning and treatment response predictions [52].

In addition, with up-to-date evidence pointing toward better survival and better visual outcomes with early treatment of JIA and JIA-uveitis, there is a worldwide tendency toward starting immunosuppressive therapy sooner rather than later. On the other hand, long-term data on potential side effects and complications of reasonably new medications, as biologics, will help us better understand the long-term impact of these, so we can provide young people and their family with more accurate information on what to expect.

Children and young people with arthritis and uveitis are increasingly seen as capable of being involved in their treatment decisions, and the mental health impacts of a chronic condition in their growth and personal development is fortunately being taken into account more frequently. The importance of multidisciplinary teams and a holistic approach on healthcare is progressively valued.

9. Conclusion and take-home messages

JIA is the most common rheumatic disease in children and adolescents. JIA-associated uveitis is, not only its most frequent extra-articular manifestation, but also the most common cause of uveitis in the pediatric population.

JIA-associated uveitis is responsible for significant personal, familiar, and economic burdens as it is usually an asymptomatic uveitis, what delays its diagnosis and, therefore, treatment. This results in an incidence of ocular complications as high as 67% in affected children. Also, unfortunately, one-third of the patients present with sight-threatening complications at the time of diagnosis.

Timely screening in children and adolescents who have suspected or recently diagnosed JIA is crucial for avoiding vision impairment and improving the health-related quality of life of JIA patients. Screening frequency is based on clinical and laboratorial risk factors for developing uveitis.

If the patient has already JIA-associated uveitis, appropriate monitoring is essential to determine the type of treatment necessary and for uveitis control. Monitoring frequency is based on the degree of AC inflammation, the response to treatment and the presence of ocular complication.

Conflict of interest

The authors declare no conflict of interest.

Author details

Luiza M. Neves[1,2*] and Marcela Bohn de A. Alves[3,4]

1 Instituto Nacional de Saúde da Mulher, da Criança e do Adolescente Fernandes Figueira, Fundação Oswaldo Cruz, Rio de Janeiro, RJ, Brazil

2 Opthalmology Department of Universidade do Estado do Rio de Janeiro, Rio de Janeiro, RJ, Brazil

3 Moorfields Eye Hospital NHS Foundation Trust, London, UK

4 West Hertfordshire Teaching Hospitals NHS Trust, London, UK

*Address all correspondence to: luiza.macneves@gmail.com

References

[1] Sen ES, Ramanan AV. Juvenile idiopathic arthritis-associated uveitis. Best Practice & Research. Clinical Rheumatology. 2017;**31**(4):34

[2] Saurenmann RK et al. Prevalence, risk factors, and outcome of uveitis in juvenile idiopathic arthritis: A long-term followup study. Arthritis and Rheumatism. 2007;**56**(2):647-657

[3] Edelsten C, Lee V, Bentley CR, Kanski JJ, Graham EM. An evaluation of baseline risk factors predicting severity in juvenile idiopathic arthritis associated uveitis and other chronic anterior uveitis in early childhood. The British Journal of Ophthalmology. 2022;**86**(1):51-56. DOI: 10.1136/bjo.86.1.51

[4] de Boer J, Rothova A. Visual loss in uveitis of childhood. The British Journal of Ophthalmology. 2003;**87**(7):5

[5] Smith JA, Sen HN, Leigh JF, Watkins AS, Pyatetsky D, Tessler HH, et al. Epidemiology and course of disease in childhood uveitis. Ophthalmology. 2009;**116**(8):8

[6] Neves LM et al. Monitoring and treatment of juvenile idiopathic arthritis-associated uveitis: Brazilian evidence-based practice guidelines. Ocular Immunology and Inflammation. 2022; **30**(6):1384-1398

[7] Heiligenhaus A et al. Review for disease of the year: Epidemiology of juvenile idiopathic arthritis and its associated uveitis: The probable risk factors. Ocular Immunology and Inflammation. 2013;**21**(3):180-191. DOI: 10.3109/09273948.2013.791701

[8] Thierry S et al. Prevalence and incidence of juvenile idiopathic arthritis: A systematic review. Joint, Bone, Spine. 2014;**81**(2):112-117

[9] Jari M et al. Epidemiological and advanced therapeutic approaches to treatment of uveitis in pediatric rheumatic diseases: A systematic review and meta-analysis. Orphanet Journal of Rare Diseases. 2020;**15**(1):41. DOI: 10.1186/s13023-020-1324-x

[10] Tay-Kearney ML, Lowder C, Dunn JP, Meisler DM, Vitale S, Jabs DA. Clinical features and associated systemic diseases of HLA-B27 uveitis. American Journal of Ophthalmology. 1996;**121**(1):9

[11] Wolf MD, Ragsdale CG. Prognostic factors in the uveitis of juvenile rheumatoid arthritis. Ophthalmology. 1987;**94**(10):6

[12] Hoyt CS. Pediatric Ophthalmology and Strabismus. 4th ed. Saunders Ltd.; 2012

[13] Haasnoot AJW, Kuiper JJW, de Boer JH. Predicting uveitis in juvenile idiopathic arthritis: From biomarkers to clinical practice. Expert Review of Clinical Immunology. 2019;**15**(6): 657-666

[14] Du L, Yang P. Immune response genes in uveitis. Ocular Immunology and Inflammation. 2009;**17**(4):8

[15] Julián K, Quartier P, Lehoang P, Bodaghi B. Uveitis related to juvenile idiopathic arthritis: Familial cases and possible genetic implication in the pathogenesis. Ocular Immunology and Inflammation. 2010;**18**(3):5

[16] Sijssens KMEA. Cytokines, chemokinesand soluble adhesion molecules in aqueous humour of

children with uveitis. Experimental Eye Research. 2007;**85**:6

[17] Nordal E, Rypdal V, Christoffersen T, Aalto K, Berntson L, Fasth A, et al. Incidence and predictors of Uveitis in juvenile idiopathic arthritis in a Nordic long-term cohort study. Pediatric Rheumatology Online Journal. 18 Aug 2017;**15**(1):66. DOI: 10.1186/s12969-017-0195-8. PMID: 28821293; PMCID: PMC5562983

[18] Saurenmann RK, Feldman BM, Laxer RM, Schneider R. Risk factors for development of uveitis differ between girls and boys with juvenile idiopathic arthritis. Arthritis and Rheumatism. 2010;**62**(6):4

[19] Chia A et al. Factors related to severe uveitis at diagnosis in children with juvenile idiopathic arthritis in a screening program. American Journal of Ophthalmology. 2003;**135**(6):757-762

[20] Heiligenhaus A, Ganser G, Heinz C, Minden K. Prevalence and complications of uveitis in juvenile idiopathic arthritis in a population-based nation-wide study in Germany: Suggested modification of the current screening guidelines. Rheumatology. 2007;**46**(6):4

[21] Sabri K, Silverman ED, Levin AV. Course, complications and outcome of juvenile arthritis-related uveitis. Journal of AAPOS. 2008;**12**:6

[22] Constantin T, Anton J, de Boer J, Czitrom-Guillaume S, Edelsten C, Gepstein R, et al. Consensus-based recommendations for the management of uveitis associated with juvenile idiopathic arthritis: The SHARE initiative. Annals of the Rheumatic Diseases. 2018;**77**(8):10

[23] Kalinina Ayuso V, van der Does P, Rothova A, de Boer JH. Male gender as a risk factor for complications in uveitis associated with juvenile idiopathic arthritis. American Journal of Ophthalmology. 2010;**149**(6):5

[24] Holland GN. Special considerations in the evaluation and management of uveitis in children. American Journal of Ophthalmology. 2003;**135**(6):11

[25] Heiligenhaus A, Föll D, Pleyer U. Uveitis in juvenile idiopathic arthritis. Deutsches Ärzteblatt International. 2015; **112**(6):8

[26] Holland GN, Yu F. Chronic anterior uveitis in children: Clinical characteristics and complications. American Journal of Ophthalmology. 2009;**147**(4):11

[27] Jhanji V, Vajpayee RB. Corneal calcific band keratopathy. Current Opinion in Ophthalmology. 2011;**22**(4):6

[28] Thorne JE, Dunn JP, Jabs DA. Risk of cataract development among children with juvenile idiopathic arthritis-related uveitis treated with topical corticosteroids. Ophthalmology. 2010; **117**(7):5

[29] Choi J, Ashworth J, Edelsten C, Bossuyt A. An update on the modern management of paediatric uveitis. The British Journal of Ophthalmology. 2019; **103**:1685-1689

[30] Esmael A, Elhusseiny AM, Fayed AE, Elhilali HM. Agreement profiles for rebound and applanation tonometry in normal and glaucomatous children. European Journal of Ophthalmology. 2019;**29**(4):379-385

[31] Moradi A, Reddy AK, Hornbeak DM, Leung TG, Burkholder BM, Thorne JE. Risk of hypotony in juvenile idiopathic arthritis-associated uveitis. American

Journal of Ophthalmology. 2016;**169**: 113-124

[32] de Boer J et al. Development of macular edema and impact on visual acuity in uveitis associated with juvenile idiopathic arthritis. Ocular Immunology and Inflammation. 2015;**23**(1):67-73

[33] Paroli MP et al. Retinal complications of juvenile idiopathic arthritis-related uveitis: A microperimetry and optical coherence tomography study. Ocular Immunology and Inflammation. 2010; **18**(1):54-59

[34] Davies K et al. BSPAR standards of care for children and young people with juvenile idiopathic arthritis. Rheumatology (Oxford). 2010;**49**(7):1406-1408

[35] The Royal College of Ophthalmologists, British Society of Paediatric and Adolescent Rheumatology Guidelines for screening for uveitis in juvenile idiopathic arthritis. 2006

[36] Angeles-Han ST et al. 2019 American College of Rheumatology/ Arthritis Foundation Guideline for the screening, monitoring, and treatment of juvenile idiopathic arthritis-associated uveitis. Arthritis Care & Research (Hoboken). 2019;**71**(6):703-716

[37] de Moraes AJPVA, Len C, et al. Projeto diretrizes: Artrite idiopática juvenil: Diagnóstico. Associação Médica Brasileira. 2012:16

[38] Jabs DA et al. Standardization of uveitis nomenclature for reporting clinical data. Results of the First International Workshop. American Journal of Ophthalmology. 2005;**140**(3): 509-516

[39] Hawkins MJ et al. Managing juvenile idiopathic arthritis-associated uveitis. Survey of Ophthalmology. 2016;**61**(2): 197-210

[40] Bou R, Borrás F, et al. Clinical management algorithm of uveitis associated with juvenile idiopathic arthritis: Interdisciplinary panel consensus. Rheumatology International. 2015;**35**:8. DOI: 10.1007/s00296-015-3231-3

[41] Heiligenhaus A, Tappeiner C, et al. Update of the evidence based, interdisciplinary guideline for anti-inflammatory treatment of uveitis associated with juvenile idiopathic arthritis. Seminars in Arthritis and Rheumatism. 2019:49

[42] Moorthy LN et al. Burden of childhood-onset arthritis. Pediatric Rheumatology. 2010;**8**(1):20

[43] Minden K, Listing J, Biedermann T, Schöntube M, Zink A. Burden and cost of illness in patients with juvenile idiopathic arthritis. Annals of the Rheumatic Diseases. 2004;**63**(7):836-842

[44] Allen T, Reda S, Martin S, Long P, Franklin A, Bedoya SZ, et al. The needs of adolescents and young adults with chronic illness: Results of a quality improvement survey. Children (Basel). 2 Apr 2022;**9**(4):500. DOI: 10.3390/ children9040500. PMID: 35455544; PMCID: PMC9025253

[45] McDonald J, Altaye M, Andringa J, Cooper AM, Drews-Botsch C, Engelhard G Jr, et al. Comprehensive assessment of quality of life, functioning, and mental health in children with juvenile idiopathic arthritis and noninfectious uveitis. Arthritis Care & Research (Hoboken). 2022;**74**(8):1311-1320

[46] Parker DM, Stanton AL, Holland GN. Chronic anterior uveitis in children: Psychosocial challenges for

patients and their families. American Journal of Ophthalmology. 2018;**191**:xvi-xxiv. DOI: 10.1016/j.ajo.2018.03.028

[47] Sophia Zagora TK, Singh-Grewal D, Chaitow J, McCluskey PJ, Grigg JR. Improving paediatric uveitis visual outcomes and quality of life. Investigative Ophthalmology & Visual Science. 2022;**63**(7):3184-A0410

[48] Angeles-Han ST. Quality-of-life metrics in pediatric uveitis. International Ophthalmology Clinics. 2015;**55**(2): 93-101

[49] Tugal-Tutkun I. Pediatric uveitis. Journal of Ophthalmic and Vision Research. 2011;**6**(4):259-269

[50] Chan NS, Choi J, Cheung CMG. Pediatric Uveitis. Asia-Pacific Journal of Ophthalmology (Phila). 2018;**7**(3): 192-199

[51] Martini A et al. Toward new classification criteria for juvenile idiopathic arthritis: First Steps, Pediatric Rheumatology International Trials Organization International Consensus. The Journal of Rheumatology. 2019; **46**(2):190-197

[52] Zaripova LN et al. Juvenile idiopathic arthritis: From aetiopathogenesis to therapeutic approaches. Pediatric Rheumatology Online Journal. 2021; **19**(1):135

Section 2

Posterior Uveitis

Chapter 4

Vogt-Koyanagi-Harada Disease: Current Diagnosis and Management

Anubhav Goyal, Vineet Shah, Giridhar Anantharaman and Mahesh Gopalakrishnan

Abstract

Vogt-Koyanagi-Harada (VKH) disease is a rare granulomatous inflammatory disease that affects pigmented structures, such as eye, inner ear, meninges, skin, and hair. This disease is mainly a T1 lymphocyte-mediated aggression to melanocytes. The availability of new investigational methods has improved our knowledge of the pathogenesis, clinical approach, diagnosis, and management of VKH disease. The disease has an acute onset of bilateral blurred vision with hyperemia in the absence of prior ocular trauma or any previous intraocular surgery. The chronic phase comprises of ocular and integumentary system pigmentary changes. Ocular findings may be accompanied by meningismus, hearing impairment, and skin lesions in a variable proportion of patients. Prompt diagnosis with early, aggressive, and long-term treatment of high-dose corticosteroids ensures good visual outcomes. The aim of this chapter is to present the clinicopathology, classification, recent imaging, investigations, and management of VKH disease.

Keywords: Vogt-Koyanagi-Harada disease, granulomatous uveitis, imaging, immunomodulatory therapy, optical coherence tomography, corticosteroids, immunosuppressant

1. Introduction

Vogt-Koyanagi-Harada (VKH) disease, formerly called as uveo-meningitic syndrome, is a systemic autoimmune disorder involving multiple organ systems, including the ocular, auditory, nervous, and integumentary. Severe bilateral panuveitis along with exudative retinal detachment is characteristic for this disease [1]. Fluorescein angiography and optical coherence tomography (OCT) have helped diagnose the condition through the analysis of changes in the retina and, recently, the choroid. Corticosteroids and, more recently, steroid-sparing immunomodulators have been the mainstay of treatment [2].

2. History

VKH disease was first described by Ali-ibn-Isa (940-1010 AD) who described inflammation of the eyes and whitening of the eyelashes, eyebrows, and hair (poliosis) [3]. In 1873, this association was reported again by Schenkl followed by Hutchinson in 1892 and Vogt in 1906 [4–6]. In 1962, the Japanese physician Einosuke Harada described a posterior uveitis accompanied by exudative retinal detachment and cerebrospinal fluid (CSF) pleocytosis [7]. In 1929, bilateral iridocyclitis associated with vitiligo, alopecia, and poliosis along with tinnitus and deafness was described by Koyanagi [8]. Babel in 1932 and later Bruno and McPherson in 1949 combined the descriptions of Vogt, Koyanagi, and Harada and proposed that these signs and symptoms were a series of manifestations of the same underlying disease process, differing only in intensity and the distribution from one patient to another [9, 10]. A common alternative to uveomeningoencephalitic syndrome is VKH disease, which has existed since then.

3. Epidemiology

While population-based epidemiological studies are relatively rare, epidemiological data from tertiary referral centers indicate a wide variation in the incidence of VKH disease. A predilection for this disease occurs among those with dark pigments, in particular Asians, Hispanics, Middle Easterners, and Native Americans [1]. Geographically, VKH syndrome accounts for an estimated 4% of all uveitis referrals in the United States and 8% in Japan [10]. These patients appear to vary globally in their gender predilection, but most studies suggest that women are affected somewhat more often than men [11–17]. Most patients are in the second to fifth decades of life at the onset of the disease and while uncommon, it has been well recognized in children [11–14, 17–22].

The most common cause of panuveitis in India is VKH, with a prevalence of 21.08% [2]. Martin and colleagues studied new cases of uveitis in South India and found that 1.2% were diagnosed with VKH, of which 8.2% were children [2]. An average age of 13.5 years was observed among patients between the ages of 8 and 16. In 75% of the cases, the final vision of the child was better than 20/40 [2].

4. Etiology and pathogenesis

There is no definitive etiology or pathogenesis for VKH syndrome, but it is believed that it is primarily the result of an autoimmune inflammatory reaction that targets melanin-containing cells or a common antigen present in the skin, eye, meninges, and ear. Following viral infection-induced challenge, an autoimmune attack against melanocyte-associated antigens is considered the most likely mechanism in genetically susceptible individuals (**Figure 1**). According to some studies, individuals who are genetically susceptible develop an autoimmune response mediated by T lymphocytes against self-antigens associated with melanocytes across all organ systems [24, 25]. Research suggests that HLA-DR4 is associated with the disease among Japanese, and HLA-DR1 or HLA-DR4 with Hispanic patients from southern California, further supporting the genetic predisposition [26, 27].

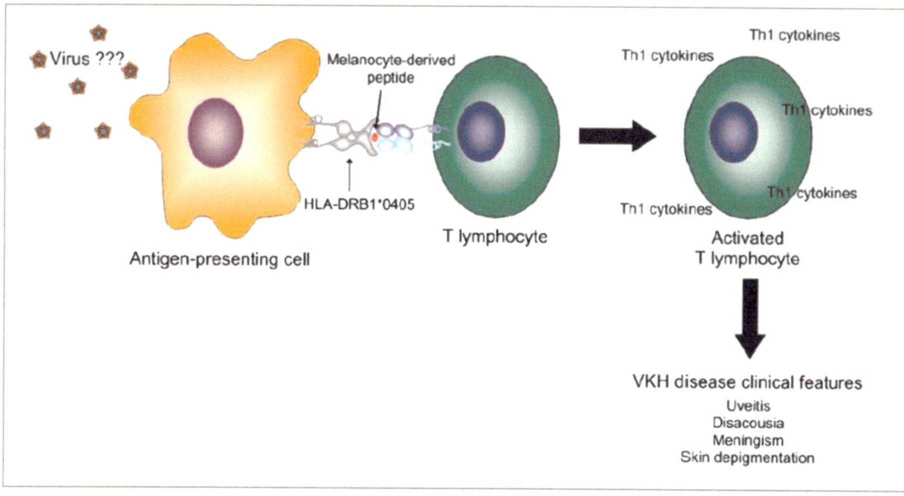

Figure 1.
Pathogenesis of VKH [23].

Studies have shown that tyrosinase protein antigens are reactive with lymphocytes of VKH patients, suggesting that these proteins are the target antigens of immune reactions in this disease. Patients with VKH disease have helper CD4+ lymphocytes in vitiligo lesions, as well as an altered ratio of CD4+/CD8+ cells (3:1). Other studies related to dermal lesions have shown that melanin-rich cells in the epidermis are eliminated and connective tissue is infiltrated by T cells, suggesting that cell-mediated immune responses are a major pillar of pathogenesis [28].

5. Histopathological features

The histopathological features of VKH vary according to the stage of the disease. Diffuse thickening of the uveal ducts (mainly in the peripapillary choroid) is the main pathologic feature of VKH [29, 30].

In the acute stage, it is important to note that there is diffuse lymphocytic infiltration with aggregates of epithelioid cells and multinucleated giant cells without any obvious choroidal necrosis. The choroidal infiltrate consists of T lymphocytes and melanocytes expressing molecules of the class II major histocompatibility complex. During acute uveitis, the subretinal fluid is made up of eosinophilic proteinaceous material. There is diffuse infiltration of lymphocytes, epithelioid histiocytes, and multinucleated giant cells, similar to features of the choroidal stromal disease [31]. Dalen-Fuchs nodules can be formed by the accumulation of hyperplastic retinal pigment epithelium (RPE), macrophages, epithelioid cells, and lymphocytes between the RPE and Bruch's membrane [32, 33]. Histopathology during convalescent stage showed non-granulomatous inflammatory cellular infiltrate with focal lymphocyte aggregates and occasional macrophages. The loss of choroidal melanocytes results in a pale and depigmented appearance of the choroid. As a result, images like "sunset glow fundus" can be enjoyed [32, 33]. In the chronic recurrent stage, granulomatous choroiditis with choriocapillary damage can be observed. In addition, a granulomatous infiltrate can be observed, with less pronounced diffuse thickening of the uvea in comparison with the acute phase. Atrophy or proliferation of RPE is often accompanied by chorioretinal adhesions. Hyperpigmented areas in atrophic patch are due to the proliferation of RPE, rarely associated with subretinal neovascularization [33]. Immunological markers like CD3 and CD20 with increased T cell involvement have been found in cases of VKH syndrome [34].

6. Clinical manifestations

VKH disease presents in four clinically distinct phases: prodromal, uveitic, convalescent, and chronic recurrent.

6.1 Prodromal stage

The prodromal period is characterized by flu-like symptoms. Systemic associations like headache, nausea, meningeal irritation, impaired hearing, tinnitus, fever, orbital pain, photophobia, and sensitivity to touch may precede ocular symptoms. Focal neurological signs, although rare, may include multiple cranial neuropathies, hemiparesis, aphasia, transverse myelitis, and ganglionitis. CSF analysis revealed lymphocytosis and normal glucose in more than 80% of patients; this observation may persist for up to 8 weeks [1, 2, 35]. Central hearing loss occurs early in the disease course in approximately 30% of patients, usually with high frequency, and usually improves within 2–3 months; however, persistent deficits may persist.

6.2 Acute uveitic stage

The acute uveitis phase begins with persistent visual impairment in both eyes 1 to 2 days after the onset of central nervous system symptoms. It is marked by bilateral granulomatous anterior uveitis, a variable degree of vitritis, thickening of the posterior choroid, edema of the optic nerve, and multiple serous retinal detachments. There are often small, cloverleaf-shaped focal serous retinal detachments around the posterior pole. However, these can coalesce into large, bullous detachments and become exudative. Fluorescein angiogram in acute uveitic stage typically shows multiple hyperfluorescent pinpoint spots merging into pools of fluorescein in the subretinal space. Profound vision loss may be seen in this stage [22]. Less commonly, mutton fat Keratic precipitates (KPs) and inflammatory iris nodules can be seen at the pupillary margin. Secondary IOP rise, anterior chamber shallowing due to ciliary edema, and/or annular choroidal detachment resulting in anterior displacement of the lens-iris septum can be rarely seen in this stage. Alternatively, IOP may be low, possibly due to ciliary shutdown. Recent confocal scans of corneal deposits have shown that non-infectious causes of uveitis (such as VKH) appear as smooth, round deposits, while infectious uveitis appears as dendritic deposits.

6.3 Convalescent stage

The recovery phase occurs after a few weeks and is characterized by the resolution of exudative retinal detachment and progressive depigmentation of the choroid, resulting in classic orange-red discoloration or twilight fundus. Small, round, inconspicuous lesions were also present in the lower peripheral fundus. Pericapillary hyperpigmentation may also be observed. The sunset-glow fundus may show focal areas of retinal hyper- or hypopigmentation. In up to 85% of Japanese patients, perilimbal vitiligo (Sugiura sign) is present, but rarely in white patients [1]. Skin changes, including vitiligo, alopecia, and graying, usually occur during the recovery phase in approximately 30% of patients and coincide with the development of fundus hypopigmentation. Usually, skin and hair changes occur late the onset of ocular inflammation, but in some cases, they can occur at the same time. Vitiligo occurs in 10 to 63% of patients, depending on ethnicity; cutaneous manifestations and other extraocular manifestations are relatively uncommon in Hispanic patients.

7. Chronic recurrent stage

The chronic relapsing phase is characterized by recurrent episodes of granulomatous anterior uveitis with keratic precipitates, posterior synechiae, iris nodules, iris depigmentation, and stromal atrophy. Recurrent posterior segment inflammation can occur but is uncommon during this stage. It is at this stage that the vision-impairing effects of chronic inflammation appear, such as posterior subcapsular cataracts, glaucoma, choroidal neovascularization (CNV), and subretinal fibrosis.

8. Extraordinary manifestations

8.1 Integumentary system

Integumentary system manifestations are seen at various stages of the disease and these vary markedly among reported series. Seventy-two percent of patients reported sensitivity to touch of the hair and skin in the prodromal stage [18]. Alopecia, poliosis, and vitiligo are all well recognized in VKH, although their reported prevalence varies from just over 10% to over 60% in published studies [13, 14]. One report suggested that Hispanic people may have a lower dermatologic involvement incidence than Asian patients [13].

8.2 Neurologic manifestations

Headache, confusion, orbital pain, and stiff neck are common symptoms of prodromal stage. In a study published by Beniz and colleagues, headaches were by far the most common neurological complaint [13]. CSF pleocytosis with predominance of lymphocytes and monocytes with normal glucose level has been found in 80% of VKH patients [11, 18]. A rare case of polymorphonuclear pleocytosis resembling infectious meningitis in VKH has also been reported earlier. Rarely, focal neurological signs such as cranial neuropathies, hemiplegia, aphasia, transverse myelitis, and ganglionitis are also associated [36–38].

8.3 Auditory manifestations

Hearing problems such as tinnitus occur in 75% of patients, often associated with active eye disease [39]. Hearing loss is usually for higher frequencies but rarely can affect all frequencies [40]. Improvement is usually seen within 2–3 months, but persistent changes may occur [18].

9. Unilateral VKH

Although bilateral involvement is required for the diagnosis of VKH according to the current revised diagnostic criteria, there have been a few reports of monocular or asymmetrical ocular involvement [41–44]. VKH may present with atypical features, such as unilateral or asymmetric signs and symptoms. Forster et al., Roe et al., and Usui et al. have reported cases of unilateral VKH or cases in which the fellow eye was involved late [41, 43, 44].

10. Diagnostic criteria

Several sets of criteria have been proposed for the diagnosis of VKH disease, since it was initially considered as a single clinical uveitis entity. The evolution of the criteria reflects our growing understanding of the disease. Diagnosis of VKH disease is straightforward and is based on suspicion of bilateral acute diffuse uveitis and various extraocular features. However, this condition may bear considerable similarity to sympathetic ophthalmia, which is also characterized by bilateral acute diffuse uveitis with alopecia, vitiligo, whitening of hair, and hearing loss. However, the latter usually occurs after ocular trauma or intraocular surgery and rarely has extraocular manifestations.

Diagnosis of VKH is primarily based on clinical features. Several criteria have been proposed to specify the diagnostic approach, including the American Uveitis Society (AUS) in 1978 (**Table 1**) and the Sugiura criteria in 1976 (**Table 2**). The AUS adopted the following diagnostic criteria [12, 29].

1. No previous ocular trauma and/or surgery;
2. At least three of the following four signs are present;
3. Bilateral chronic iridocyclitis;
4. Posterior uveitis (multifocal exudative retinal or RPE detachments; disc hyperemia or edema; or "sunset glow fundus," which is a yellow-orange appearance of the fundus due to depigmentation of the RPE and choroid);
5. Neurologic signs (tinnitus, neck stiffness, cranial nerve or central nervous system symptoms, or cerebral spinal fluid pleocytosis);
6. Cutaneous signs (alopecia, poliosis, or vitiligo).

1. Patient should have no history of ocular trauma or surgery
2. At least three of the following four signs should be present: a. Bilateral chronic iridocyclitis, b. Posterior uveitis, including exudative retinal detachment, forme fruste of exudative retinal detachment, disk hyperemia or edema, and "sunset glow" fundus, c. Neurologic signs of tinnitus, neck stiffness, cranial nerve or central nervous system problems, or CSF pleocytosis d. Cutaneous findings of alopecia, poliosis, or vitiligo.
[a] *From Snyder and Tessler, 1980.*

Table 1.
Criteria proposed by the American Uveitis Society for diagnosis of VKH disease.

Major Symptoms
1. Acute bilateral uveitis with simultaneous involvement of both eyes. Symptoms may not be noted for 1–10 days in the second eye. 2. Circumscribed retinal edema most markedly at the posterior pole. Fluorescein angiography reveals characteristic leakage of dye through the retinal pigment epithelium into the subretinal spaces. 3. Pleocytosis of the cerebrospinal fluid is noted in the early stages of the disease. Dysacousia, vertigo, and scalp sensitivity when touching the hair are of value in early diagnosis, if present.
Minor symptoms
1. Floating cells in the anterior chamber, granulomatous keratic precipitates, and iris nodules are important signs that may be absent in early stages. 2. Hair loss and depigmentation of the eye, skin, and hair are also important signs in the convalescent stage. Depigmentation of the corneal limbus (Sugiura's sign) appears earliest (Friedman and Deutsch-Sokol, 1981), roughly 1 month after onset, and is also of value for confirming the early diagnosis if present.

Table 2.
Diagnostic criteria proposed by Sugiura for VKH disease (Sugiura, 1978).

The AUS criteria fail to distinguish acute from chronic cases. Another limitation consists of the inadequate compilation of acute cases, as two of the four cardinal signs characteristically occur in the convalescent/chronic stages of the disease. AUS criteria failed to consider fluorescein (FA), indocyanine angiography (ICGA), and ultrasonographic findings. Therefore, neither chronological examinations nor extra examinations were taken into account.

Sugiura et al. proposed another set of diagnostic criteria for VHK (**Table 2**). This system is seldom used outside Japan, where CSF analysis is mandatory [12, 22]. Sugiura's criteria included 3 main symptoms: simultaneous bilateral uveitis, localized retinal edema at the posterior pole with characteristic fluorescent dye leakage, and pleocytosis of CSF in acute phase. According to Sugiura's criteria, CSF pleocytosis is also an important sign necessary for the diagnosis of the disease [2]. The International Nomenclature Committee defined more comprehensive criteria, the Revised Diagnostic Criteria (RDC) in 2001 [30]. RDC divides the disease into three categories based on the presence of extraocular findings: complete, incomplete, and probable VKH (**Table 3**) [30]. By considering both early and late ocular manifestations, patients can be diagnosed regardless of time since presentation. Additional examinations (i.e., ICGA and optical coherence tomography (OCT) were not considered. RDC also did not consider follow-up period and treatment; these two parameters can interfere with the occurrence of extraocular manifestations.

More recently, a correlation between fundus changes and full-field electroretinogram (ffERG) with advanced VKH (more than 6 months after onset) was shown by da Silva et al. Fundus parameters were used to provide a framework for analyzing fundus changes in advanced stages of VKH, namely: diffuse pigmentary changes; nummular lesions; pigmented masses; and subretinal fibrosis [45]. Correlations of severity in fundus with ffERG parameters suggest that fundus changes may reflect functional abnormalities. Lumbar puncture is helpful only for diagnosing acute VKH. Given the large number of patients with hearing problems, audiometry is recommended in patients with VKH [35].

11. Diagnosis

The diagnosis of VKH is clinical (as no laboratory marker identifies the presence thereof) and is based on the RDC to date (**Table 3**) [30]. It is common trend in the United States and several other countries for most patients to undergo retinal fluorescein angiography if VKH has been suspected. Japanese and European doctors perform lumbar punctures to detect pleocytosis in cerebrospinal fluid. A variety of other investigations may be useful in identifying VKH, including indocyanine green (ICG)

Complete Vogt-Koyanagi-Harada disease (criteria 1 to 5 must be present)
1. No history of penetrating ocular trauma or surgery preceding the initial onset of uveitis. 2. No clinical or laboratory evidence suggestive of other ocular disease entities. 3. Bilateral ocular involvement (A or B must be met): a. Early manifestations of disease 1. Diffuse choroiditis (with or without anterior uveitis, vitreous reaction, or optic disk hyperemia), as manifested by either: a. Focal areas of subretinal fluid, or b. Bullous serous retinal detachments 2. With equivocal fundus findings, both of the following must be present as well: a. Focal area of delay in choroidal perfusion, multifocal areas of pinpoint leakage, large placoid areas of hyperfluorescence, pooling within subretinal fluid, and optic nerve staining (listed in order of sequential appearance) by fluorescein angiography, and b. Diffuse choroidal thickening, without evidence of posterior scleritis by ultrasonography. b. Late manifestations of disease 1. History suggestive of prior presence of findings from IIIA, and either both 2 and 3 below, or multiple signs from 3. 2. Ocular depigmentation (either of the following manifestations is sufficient): a. Sunset glow fundus, or b. Sugiura signs 3. Other ocular signs a. Nummular chorioretinal depigmented scars, or b. Retinal pigment epithelium clumping and/or migration, or c. Recurrent or chronic anterior uveitis. 4. Neurological/auditory findings (may have resolved by time of examination). a. Meningismus (malaise, fever, headache, nausea, abdominal pain, stiffness of the neck and back) or b. Tinnitus, or c. Cerebrospinal fluid pleocytosis 5. Integumentary finding (not preceding onset of central nervous system or ocular disease) a. Alopecia, or b. Poliosis, or c. Vitiligo
Incomplete Vogt-Koyanagi-Harada disease (criteria 1 to 3 and either 4 or 5 must be present)
1. No history of penetrating ocular trauma or surgery preceding the initial onset of uveitis, and 2. No clinical or laboratory evidence suggestive of other ocular disease entities, and 3. Bilateral ocular involvement, and, either 4. Neurologic/auditory findings; as defined for complete Vogt-Koyanagi-Harada disease above, or 5. Integumentary findings; as defined for complete Vogt-Koyanagi-Harada disease above
Probable Vogt-Koyanagi-Harada disease (isolated ocular disease: criteria 1 to 3 must be present)
1. No history of penetrating ocular trauma or surgery preceding the initial onset of uveitis. 2. No clinical or laboratory evidence suggestive of other ocular disease entities. Bilateral ocular involvement as defined for complete Vogt-Koyanagi-Harada disease above. Isolated ocular disease.
[a] *From Am J Ophthalmol 2001:131, 647-652.*

Table 3.
Revised diagnostic criteria for Vogt-Koyanagi-Harada Disease.

angiography and ultrasonography, which measure choroidal thickness. However, although electroretinograms and electroencephalograms have been used in the past, these procedures are rarely conducted and may not be necessary for diagnosing VKH in the vast majority of cases. Recent advances in imaging technology have made it possible not only to analyze but also to objectively evaluate disease progression and treatment efficacy in VKH patients (**Table 4**). Advances in OCT in the measurement of choroidal thickness, along with other imaging modalities, have enabled the non-invasive delineation of changes in the retina, retinal pigment epithelium, and choroid that were previously not apparent on clinical examination [2].

11.1 Fluorescein angiography (FA)

Changes in FA during the acute uveitic stage are characteristic and can help differentiate VKH from other conditions. Initially, in the setting of active inflammation, FA showed delayed choroidal perfusion, resulting in hypofluorescence in poorly perfused areas. There are numerous consecutive hyperfluorescent pinpoint spots, possibly corresponding to alterations in the RPE. When these hyperfluorescent spots magnify and stain the surrounding subretinal fluid, a pool of stain appears in the subretinal space. The areas of choroiditis correspond to these hyperfluorescent lesions. During the acute phase of the disease, nearly 70% of patients develop disc leaks (**Figures 2–4**) [47]. Some linear areas of hypofluorescence can be observed due to the presence of choroidal ischemia or folds. The presence and extent of the pinpoint leakage can be used to monitor the effectiveness of initial treatment with corticosteroids. During the recovery phase, disc leaks and hyperfluorescent spots were also observed in 29% and 14% of patients, respectively [48, 49].

In the chronic and recurrent stages, FA may exhibit multiple hyperfluorescent window defects, as well as areas of blocked hypofluorescence in areas of damaged RPE, presenting as "moth-eaten" appearance. Choroidal neovascularization (CNV), retinochoroidal anastomosis, and disc neovascularization may be seen rarely [35].

11.2 Indocyanine green angiography (ICGA)

ICGA is commonly used for studying inflammatory pathologies of choroidal vasculature and stroma [50]. Herbert et al. reviewed and described characteristic ICGA signs in VKH disease. Inflammatory damage to choroidal vessels can lead to delayed choroidal perfusion in the early stages of ICGA (2–3 minutes after dye injection) [48, 51, 52]. Even when fundus and FA findings are inconspicuous, hypofluorescent spots may appear in the early stages of ICGA; thus, ICGA can serve as a sensitive marker for the detection and monitoring of subclinical choroidal inflammation (**Figure 4**). The heterogeneous background choroidal fluorescence observed at provisional ICGA is the result of multiple hypofluorescent circular lesions in the choroidal stroma (**Figures 2–4**). Early hyperfluorescence with leakage throughout the choroidal stroma along with loss of large choroidal vessels (dark vessels) in intermediate stages causes diffuse hyperfluorescence. Numerous hypofluorescent and homogeneous lesions (black dots) in the intermediate stage gradually become isofluorescent in the late stage signifies choroidal granulomas (**Figure 2**). Optic disc hyperfluorescence can also be seen in late phase.

Until recently, disease activity parameters in non-acute VKH were primarily clinical; nowadays, there is a trend toward posterior segment imaging to see signs of inflammation, as an indicator for considering systemic therapy [35].

Imaging	Initial phase	Convalescent phase	Prognosis	Role of differential diagnosis
Optical Coherence Tomography	• Exudative retinal detachment • Presence of typical fibrinous septa dividing the subretinal space into several compartments • Folds of the RPE without retinal pigment epithelial detachments • Undulations of the inner retinal layers • Markedly thickened choroid	• Progressive subfoveal choroidal thinning • Loss of small choroidal vessels with stromal scarring • Thinning of RPE layers and disruption of outer retinal layers in the area of RPE atrophy • Progressive posterior bowing on OCT during the follow-up period	• The eyes with RPE undulations were more likely to develop posterior recurrences and have worse vision at 12 months	• Differential diagnosis with acute bilateral central serous chorioretinopathy with multiple retinal pigment epithelial detachments
Fundus Autofluorescence	• Hyperautofluorescence in the macula mixed with hypoautofluorescence in the areas of serous retinal detachment • (mild and uniform pattern if presented within 1 week after onset, diffuse and mottled pattern for delayed presentation) [46]	• Scattered and widespread hyperautofluorescence, which gradually became evident and concentrated in the macula, partially resulting in some hypoautofluorescent dots at 6 months	• Non-invasive imaging helps accessing granular hyperautofluorescence in eyes with acute and/or persistent inflammation.	NA
Fundus Fluorescein Angiography	• Focal areas of delay in choroidal perfusion • Multifocal punctuate hyperfluorescent at the level of RPE • Pooling of dye within subretinal space in areas of neurosensory detachment, and • Optic disc head staining	• Multiple hyperfluorescent window defects without progressive staining in areas of focal RPE loss and atrophy. • Absent optic disc fluorescence	• The absence of early pinpoint peripapillary hyperfluorescence on pretreatment FFA is a poor prognostic factor for developing chronic VKH	• For atypical cases without clinically evident exudative retinal detachment, FFA revealed optic disc hyperfluorescence corresponding to bilateral optic disc swelling in 97% of eyes.
Indocyanine Green Angiography	• Delayed choroidal perfusion • Early choroidal stromal vessel hyperfluorescence and leakage	• Decreased choroidal stromal hyperfluorescence and disc hyperfluorescence	• Hypofluorescent dark dots and fuzziness of stromal vessel is sign of persisting activity • Early hyperfluorescent choroidal vessels and disc hyperfluorescence	• For atypical cases without clinically evident exudative retinal detachment, ICGA disclosed decreases in the number of large choroidal vessels and fuzzy

DOI: http://dx.doi.org/10.5772/intechopen.111594

Imaging	Initial phase	Convalescent phase	Prognosis	Role of differential diagnosis
	• Hypofluorescent dark dots (HDD) during the intermediate phase, • Intermediate to late fuzzy vascular pattern and, • Optic disc hyperfluorescence		are indicative of more acute disease. • Thus, ICGA can be a sensitive marker of monitoring subclinical inflammation	choroidal vessels in more than 97% of eyes
Ultrasound Biomicroscopy	• Ciliary body edema with ciliochoroidal detachment • Shallow anterior chamber • Acute angle closure	• Ciliary thickness and area significantly increased in the recurrent group compared with the initial-onset group • Absence of ciliochoroidal detachment	NA	• Distinguish between angle closure in these eyes arising from ciliary edema rather from a primary angle-closure mechanism
B-scan Ultrasonography	• Diffuse, low- to medium-reflective choroidal thickening, predominating around optic nerve head • Serous retinal detachment, located inferiorly or in the • Posterior pole • Mild vitreous opacities • Thickening of the sclera and/or episclera posteriorly	• The amount of choroidal and scleral thickening, as well as the degree of serous elevation of the retina, decreased significantly after several weeks of therapy	NA	• Indicated for a typical presentation or with poor fundus visualization. • Differential diagnosis with posterior scleritis, where the scleral thickening has high reflectivity and is frequently accompanied by "I" sign—some of the characteristic features may be either absent or difficult to visualize in the presence of opaque media

Table 4.
Multimodal imaging in VKH, clinical findings, prognostic signs, and role of differential diagnosis.

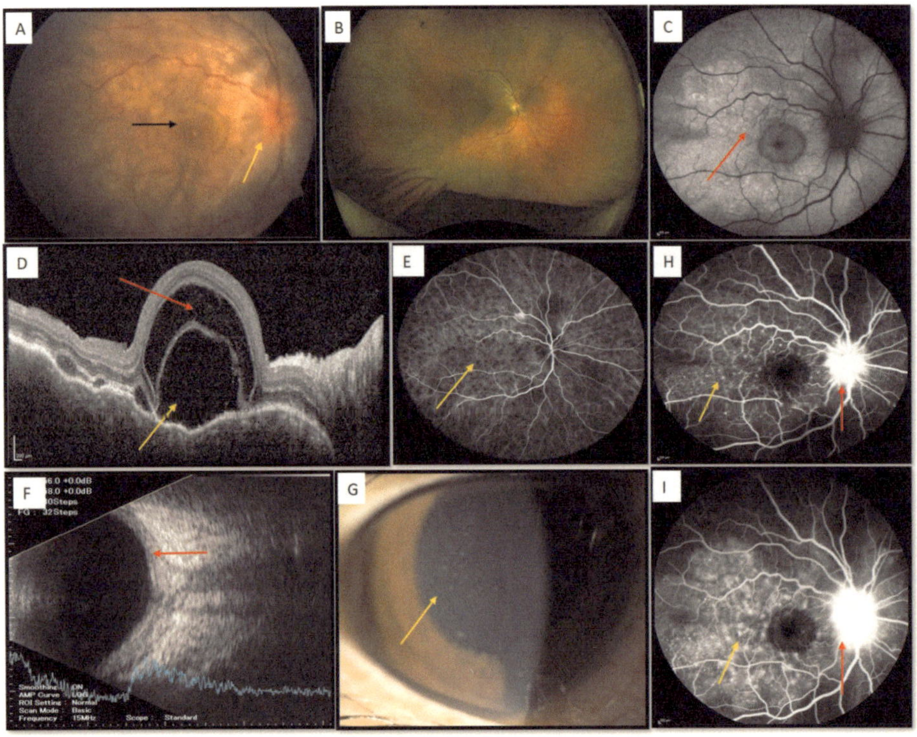

Figure 2.
Multimodal Imaging in VKH. (A) - Colour Fundus Photo shows SRF pocket (black arrow) with hyperemic disc (yellow arrow), (B) - Ultra widefield Optos Imaging showing "Sunset Glow Fundus", (C) - Fundus autofluorescence shows puntate hyperautofluorescence (red arrow), (D) - OCT shows SRF(yellow arrow) with bacillary layer detachment (red arrow) and choroidal undulations with increased choroidal thickness and obscured choroidal vessel details, (E) - ICGA showing hypofluorescence dots (yellow arrow), (F) - B scan ultrasonography showing increase in Retinal-Choroidal Scleral Complex (red arrow), (G) - Slit lamp photo showing granulomatous KPs (yellow arrow), (H & I) - Sequential fundus fluorescein angiogram (FFA) showing pinpoint hyperfluorescence (yellow arrow) increasing in late phases with pooling of dye in late phase (I) - with disc leakage (red arrow).

11.3 Fundus autofluorescence (FAF)

FAF reflects functional changes in RPE by visualizing lipofuscin or melanin or its compounds. Acute VKH shows hypoautofluorescence in areas corresponding to serous macular detachment. After subretinal fluid resolution, FAF showed hyperautofluorescence in the macular and peripapillary area corresponding to hypofluorescence on ICGA [53]. In patients treated with a first pulse of corticosteroids, areas of hyperautofluorescence disappear, whereas in patients who received delayed treatment, hyperautofluorescence persists, signifying changes in melanin distribution and lipofuscin [53]. In a retrospective study of 10 patients with chronic VKH using an ultra-wide-angle FAF, Heussen et al. demonstrated that peripheral changes in FAF images were inconsistent with color images [54]. VKH affects both the choroid and the RPE, so different FAF patterns are common.

11.4 Optical coherence tomography (OCT)

OCT has revealed the special feature of multifocal serous retinal detachments in acute VKH, with cystic spaces and membranous structures continuous to the ellipsoid

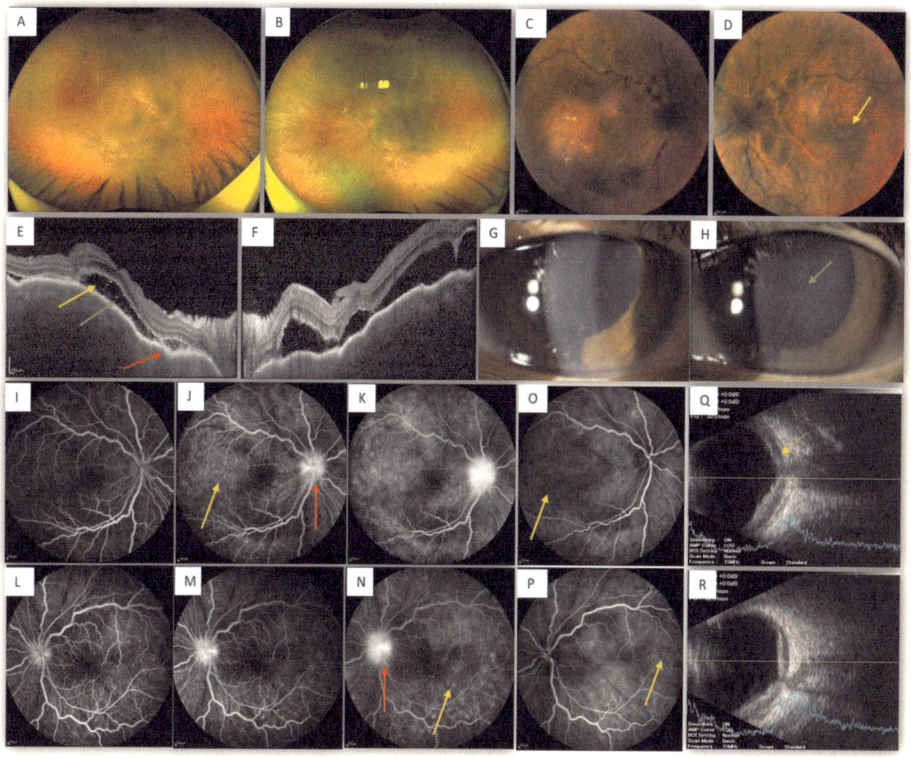

Figure 3.
Imaging in a case of bilateral VKH in a young 34 years old female. (A and B) – Ultra-wide-field Optos coloured fundus photo showing multiple SRF pockets with disc edema in right eye (A) and left eye (B), (C and D) - Multicolour image showing multiple SRF pockets with disc edema in both eyes (green arrow), (E and F) - Enhanced depth imaging EDI OCT showing subretinal fluid (yellow arrow), hyperreflective dots (green arrow), choroidal undulation with increased choroidal thickness with obscured choroidal details (red arrow) in both eyes. (G and H) – Slitlamp photo showing diffuse granulomatous KP (green arrow) in both eyes. (I,J,K,L,M,N) Fundus fluorescein angiogram (FFA) showing multiple pinpoint hyper fluorescence (yellow arrow) with disc leakage (red arrow) increasing over time from early to late phase (I- K – right eye, L-N – left eye), (O and P) Indocyanine green angiogram (ICGA) showing diffuse hypo fluorescence due to blockage of choroidal fluorescence (yellow arrow), (Q and R) B scan Ultrasound of right eye (Q) and left eye (R) showing increase in retinal–choroidal–scleral complex with subretinal exudation yellow (arrow).

zone (junction of the internal and external segments of the photoreceptors). About 45% of the examined eyes showed a splitting of retinal layers along the IS/OS line near cystoid spaces involving the fovea. All of these abnormal features were seen below the external limiting membrane, that is, in the outer photoreceptor layer [55]. Several authors hypothesized that these threads are formed by fibrin and disrupted outer segments of the photoreceptors. Many studies have also shown the presence of "bacillary layer detachment" which is defined as a separation of the retinal photoreceptor layer into the myoid inner layer and ellipsoid outer layer, as a feature of acute VKH (**Figures 2** and **4**). Other OCT findings in the acute stage are intraretinal edema, multiple subretinal fluid pockets, choroidal folds (RPE undulations), and choroidal hyperreflective dots among others (**Figures 2–4**) [55]. Rapid resolution is observed in OCT after high-dose systemic corticosteroids [56]. Several OCT parameters were associated with a worse prognosis, such as "separation" of the outer segment and inner segment of the photoreceptors, the height of the serous retinal detachment, and RPE undulation [57].

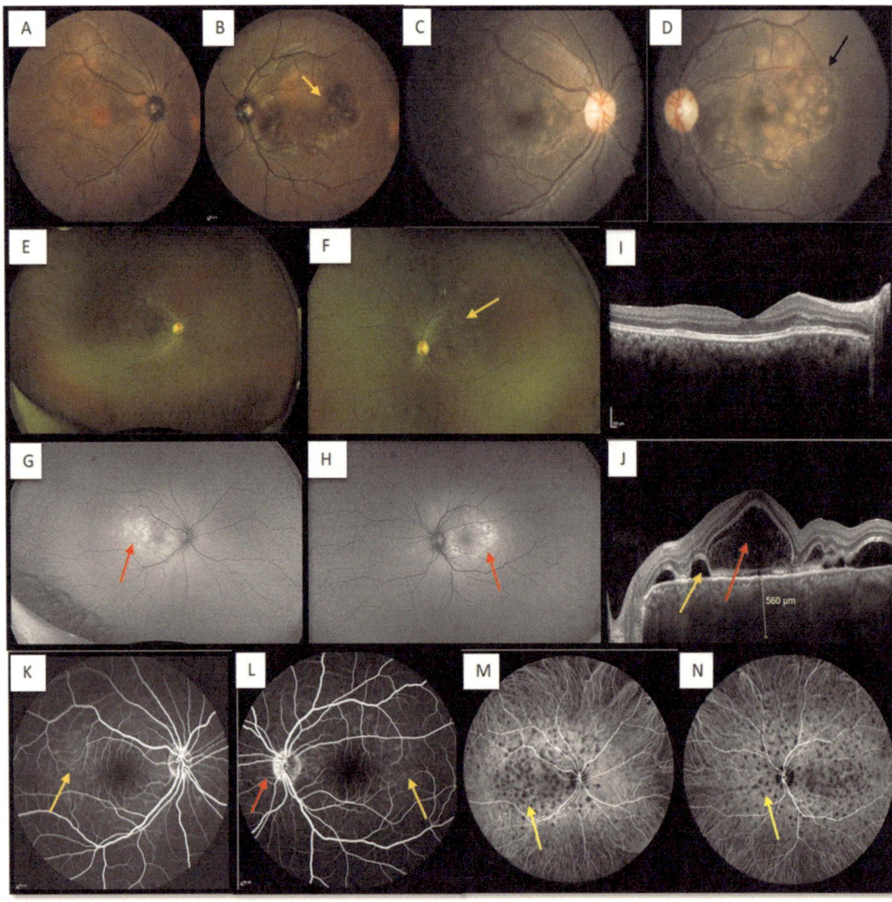

Figure 4.
Imaging of Unilateral (left eye) VKH. (A and B) Multicolour Imaging showing SRF pockets (yellow arrow) in Left Eye, (C and D) Fundus Photo showing multiple orangish lesions and SRF pockets (black arrow) in left eye, (E and F) Ultra widefield optos image showing multiple altered pigmented dots in macula of left eye (yellow arrow). (G and H) – Fundus Auto Fluorescence (FAF) showing hyperautofluorescence in both eyes (red arrow) documenting the importance of FAF in detecting changes even in very early phase of disease like in the right eye. (I and J) OCT image showing bacillary layer detachment (red arrow) and SRF pockets (yellow arrows) in left eye with increased choroidal thickness and normal retinal layers in right eye, (K and L) Fundus fluorescein angiogram (FFA) images showing disc hyperfluorescence (yellow arrow) with pin point hyper fluorescence (red arrow) in left eye, (M and N) Indocyanine green angiogram (ICGA) shows multiple hypo-fluorescent dots (yellow arrows) in both eyes documenting importance of ICGA in detecting changes even in very early phase of disease like in right eye.

OCT imaging of chronic VKH shows RPE cell clumping and damage to inner and outer photoreceptor-segment junctions. Patients with chronic VKH and "sunset glow" fundus have been studied by Vasconcelos-Santos et al. who revealed normal retinal architecture in the "sunset fundus" region, thinning of the RPE/Bruch membrane in the atrophic regions, and thickening of the RPE/Bruch membrane covering the pigmented scar regions on spectral-domain OCT [58].

11.5 Enhanced-depth imaging spectral-domain OCT (EDIOCT)

EDI-OCT is a non-invasive quantitative method that can be used to determine the extent of the choroidal inflammatory response during follow-up [58].

This modality has improved our ability to visualize the choroid and its thickness [58]. Choroidal thickening is marked in acute phase with increased inflammatory infiltrates and exudates (**Figures 2** and **4**). Corticosteroid therapy rapidly reduces choroidal thickening. According to Da Silva et al., in patients with long-term VKH, the choroid is thinner than normal counterparts [45, 60]. Additionally, the choroid is thicker in patients with recurrent inflammation compared to individuals with quiescent disease [60]. The thinning of the choroid in the center of the fovea was inversely proportional to the duration of the disease.

11.6 Ocular ultrasonography (US)

Ultrasound can be an important adjunct to diagnosis, as it can differentiate posterior scleritis, diffuse malignant melanoma, leukemia, and lymphoma [61]. It is useful when media opacity obscures fundus view, appearance is abnormal, and/or extraocular signs are absent. High-resolution ocular ultrasound can demonstrate choroidal thickening in subclinical VKH and can also help monitor treatment response. However, due to its image resolution (100 μm versus 7 μm in SD-OCT and 5 μm in EDI-OCT), US imaging does not add much information where subtle changes occur. The following sonographic signs have been described in VKH by Forster et al. [61]:

1. Diffuse choroidal thickening with low to moderate reflectivity;

2. Serous retinal detachments around or below the posterior pole;

3. Vitreous opacities without posterior vitreous detachment (PVD);

4. Scleral or episcleral thickening.

Ultrasound biomicroscopy (UBM) helps in the detailed evaluation of the ciliary body and iris. Anterior chamber shallowing can occur acutely due to ciliochoroidal detachment and ciliary body thickening. This can lead to anterior displacement of the iris-lens diaphragm, simulating acute angle-closure glaucoma [62].

11.7 Electrophysiological testing

It is helpful to monitor the course of the disease as well as demonstrate the extent of functional compromise resulting from inflammatory damage to retinal components using electroretinograms (ERGs) [63, 64]. ERG abnormalities have been described in VKH patients with extensive chorioretinal atrophy. Correlations between fundus changes and ffERG in patients with late stage VKH were nicely demonstrated by DaSilva et al. [45]. Patients with more severe fundus-based disease presented more severe retinal dysfunction [45]. As a result, both scotopic and photopic amplitudes are diffusely diminished, but implicit times remain unchanged [45].

12. Differential diagnosis

12.1 Sympathetic ophthalmia

Sympathetic ophthalmia is an autoimmune condition usually seen after penetrating trauma or surgery to the eye, exposing ocular uveal tissue molecules as antigenic material leading to the immune system-mediated inflammatory response. This condition may cause bilateral non-necrotizing granulomatous uveitis (**Table 5**) [65, 66].

12.2 Choroidal melanoma

Choroidal melanoma may present with serous retinal detachments, and non-pigmented melanomas may appear as subretinal pigmentary loss which is also seen in VKH [65, 67–69].

12.3 Infectious posterior uveitis

Syphilis, tuberculosis, and endogenous endophthalmitis may manifest as subretinal nodules, intraocular inflammation, and serous retinal detachment mimicking VKH [70, 71]. It is necessary to exclude infectious etiologies before starting immunosuppressive therapy to prevent the worsening of the disease.

12.4 Alport and cogan syndromes

Alport syndrome and Cogan syndrome may manifest as bilateral auditory abnormalities and retinal manifestations. Alport syndrome shows choroidal thickening and significant inner retinal changes. Cogan syndrome is characterized by retinal vasculitis without any subretinal changes [72, 73].

Sympathetic ophthalmia	Previous penetrating ocular trauma or intraocular surgery
Non-infectious choroiditis	Acute posterior multifocal placoid pigmentepitheliopathy (APMPPE) Birdshot chorioretinopathy Multifocal choroiditis and panuveitis (MCP) Multiple evanescent white dot syndrome (MEWDS)
Infectious choroiditis	Syphilis Tuberculosis
Other inflammatory disorders	Posterior scleritis Sarcoidosis Lupus choroidopathy
Non-inflammatory disorders	Hypertensive choroidopathy Bilateral diffuse melanocytic hyperplasia Uveal effusion syndrome Specific hypertensive illness of gestation
Masquerade syndrome	Carcinoma Leukemia Lymphoma Metastasis

Table 5.
Differential diagnosis of Vogt-Koyanagi-Harada disease.

12.5 Sarcoidosis

Sarcoidosis is the distinct cause of posterior uveitis, demonstrating periphlebitis and "candle wax dripping" on fluorescein angiography, thus differentiating it from VKH [74].

12.6 Systemic lupus erythematosus chorioretinopathy

Serous retinal detachments may be present in lupus choroidopathy, but the absence of choroidal thickening with specific systemic features helps in differentiating this disease [75].

13. Treatment

The acute stage of VKH syndrome responds to early and aggressive corticosteroid treatment. Initial dosages of high dose oral or intravenous corticosteroids are standard dosage regime without any significant difference in visual acuity outcomes or the

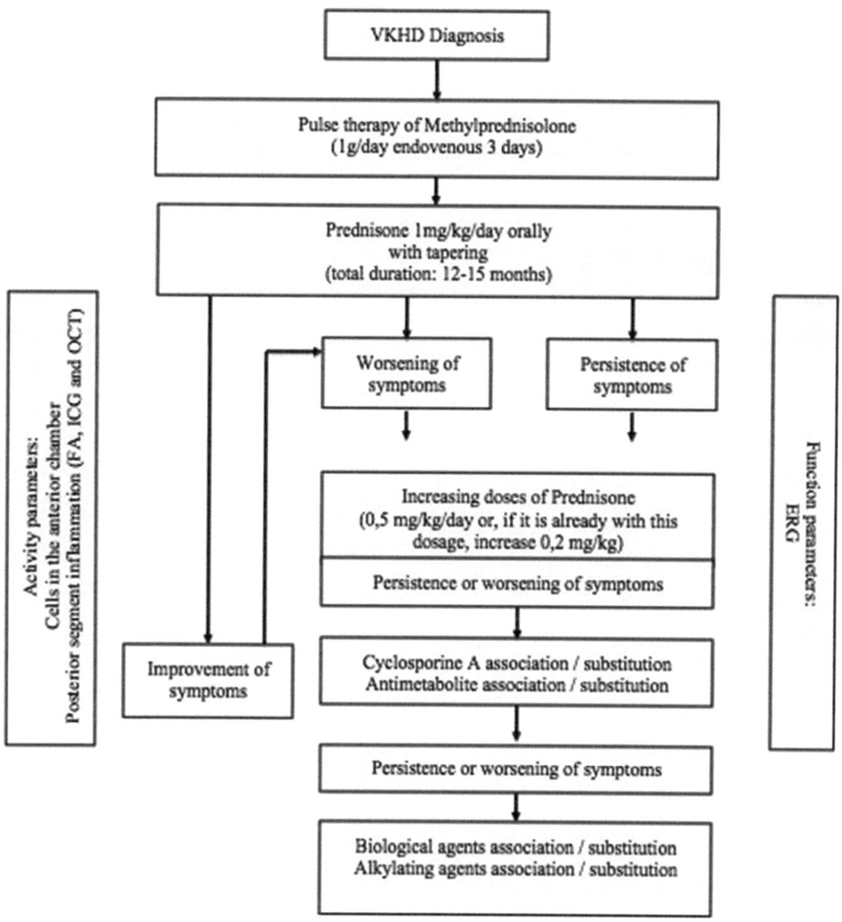

Figure 5.
Schematic flowchart for treatment protocol.

Drug	Dosage	Main side effects
Prednisone or prednisolone	1–1.5 mg/kg/day, gradual tapering along a minimum 6 month-period	Hyperglycemia, hypertension, osteoporosis, Cushingoid appearance, myopathy, cataract, glaucoma
Pulse therapy of methylprednisolone	1 g/day during 3 days, followed by oral prednisone	
Antimetabolites		
Azathioprine	1–2.5 mg/kg/day	Myelosuppression, gastrointestinal disturbances, infection
Methotrexate	7.5–25 mg/week	Nausea, vomiting, abnormalities in liver function tests, infection
Mycophenolate mofetil	1–3 g/day	gastrointestinal disturbances with diarrhea, infection
Calcineurin inhibitors		
Cyclosporine A	Up to 5 mg/kg/day, trough 0.1–0.2 μg/L (whole blood)	Nephrotoxicity, heptatoxicity, hyperglycemia, hypertension, hirsutism, gum hyperplasia, and neurological disorders
Biological agents		
Infliximab (intravenous)	5 mg/kg at 0.2 and 6 weeks, followed by 5 mg/kg every 6–8 weeks	reactivation of latent tuberculosis, lymphoproliferative diseases
Adalimumab (Subq)	40 mg every other week	Headache, infection
Alkylating agents		
Cyclophosphamide	1–2 mg/kg/day	Myelosupression, hair loss, nausea, vomiting, loss of fertility, cancer risk, infection, bladder toxicity

Table 6.
Treatment of Vogt-Koyanagi-Harada disease: drugs, dosage, and main side effects.

development of visually significant complications. Initiating immunosuppressant medication earlier can achieve more prompt inflammatory control (**Figure 5**). Slow tapering of systemic steroid along with immunosuppressants can significantly reduce chance of recurrent episodes (**Table 6**).

13.1 Systemic treatment

13.1.1 Corticosteroids

Systemic high dose corticosteroids are still the cornerstone of initial treatment for VKH. Treatment usually begins with early, high-dose systemic corticosteroids, which has a very good response. These are tapered slowly, usually over 6 months. In severe cases, some have treated with intravenous high-dose pulsed steroid therapy (1 mg of methylprednisolone) followed by oral steroids (1 mg/kg/day). Duration of treatment and rate of drug tapering are case-specific, depending on the clinical response (as shown in flowchart of **Figure 5**). Despite apparent control of clinical signs, suboptimal treatment during the post-acute period is associated with persistent choroidal inflammation. Many studies have suggested that the use of steroids for a longer duration with slow tapering prevents the reactivation of disease. Associated anterior segment inflammation should also be treated with topical prednisolone 1% and cycloplegic drugs to lessen inflammation and to reduce pain and synechiae. Topical steroids should be tapered according to the response [2].

13.1.2 Immunomodulatory therapy

Despite adequate treatment with systemic corticosteroids, many patients experience recurring episodes of inflammation and structural complications. Likewise, chronic corticosteroid therapy is associated with systemic and ocular complications. As a result, many uveitis specialists prescribe non-steroidal immunomodulatory therapy (IMT) to treat VKH at the onset of the disease, both as steroid sparing therapy and to prevent recurrence of disease. Presumably, early and aggressive immunosuppressive therapy will prevent the autoimmune process, the so-called primary reaction, and will also have a significant effect on refractory uveitis. The use of immunomodulatory therapy is associated with a reduced risk of vision loss in eyes with VKH.

Immunomodulatory therapy used in the management of VKH has been recommended as follows (**Table 6**).

- Cyclophosphamide 1–2 mg/kg/day.
- Chlorambucil 0.1–0.2 mg/kg/day.
- Azathioprine 1–2.5 mg/kg/day.
- Cyclosporine 5 mg/kg/day.
- Tacrolimus (FK 506) 0.1–0.15 mg/kg/day.
- Mycophenolate mofetil 2 mg/day.

This disease may have an immunopathologic basis in T cell-mediated damage to melanocytes as discussed previously. Several studies support the use of cyclosporine in refractory cases, either alone or with low-dose steroids [2].

13.1.3 Biologic agents

In the treatment of VKH, the main biologic agents are anti-TNF-α drugs. Several case series have reported excellent results with infliximab. Adalimumab, a human monoclonal antibody against TNF-α, has been used in refractory cases. Daclizumab, a humanized monoclonal antibody directed against the IL-2 (CD25) receptor, has shown potential in a number of reports for the treatment of non-infectious intermediate and posterior uveitis [2].

13.2 Local drug delivery

The disease is multi-organ inflammatory, so local treatment alone is not recommended. Such treatment will not eliminate the extraocular manifestations, particularly meningismus and tinnitus. Further, local treatment will not affect the severity of vitiligo or polio [2].

Topical steroids and cycloplegics are used commonly as first-line agents. Topical mydriatics and cycloplegics are used to prevent ciliary spasm and also to break and prevent the formation of posterior synechiae. Topical corticosteroid drops are most often used for anterior uveitis, but may also be beneficial in patients with panuveitis. When inflammation is severe, the hourly dosage is advised and tapering down to once a day as the inflammation improves. Topical steroid medication is associated with side effects such as ocular hypertension and the development of cataracts. Some topical preparations, such as fluorometholone 0.1%, rimexolone 1%, and loteprednol etabonate 0.5%/0.2%, have lower side effects than prednisolone acetate 1% and dexamethasone 0.1% and difluprednate 0.05%; however, the latter drugs are more effective in controlling anterior uveitis [2].

Local steroids in the form of intravitreal or subtenon injections are useful adjuncts to oral and immunosuppressive therapy. Fluocinolone acetonide (Retisert) implants have been used in chronic VKH and appear to reduce the amount of oral corticosteroids needed to control ocular inflammation, but effectiveness of oral corticosteroids could not be completely eliminated. Dexamethasone (Ozurdex) implant has also been used as alternative with successful control of refractory uveitis in some patients [2].

14. Complications

VKH complications include cataract in 15–45% of eyes, glaucoma in 27–33% of eyes, posterior synechiae in 23.4% of eyes, choroidal neovascular membrane in 3–11% of eyes. In rare instances, subretinal fibrosis (6%) and band keratopathy (5.2%) can also be seen [1].

14.1 Cataract

Steroid therapy for longer than 6 months and chronic recurrent anterior segment inflammation appeared to be the significant determinants of cataract development [1]. Cataract extraction should only be done after the uveitis has completely been treated and eye has been quiet for at least 3 months. Preoperative oral and topical corticosteroids should be started. Postoperatively, slow tapering of steroids and the use of topical NSAID drops to control cystoid macular edema are recommended [2].

14.2 Glaucoma

Acute angle closure glaucoma has been reported, presumably as a result of ciliary body edema with anterior displacement of the lens-iris diaphragm in the acute stage of the disease. The risk of developing open-angle glaucoma secondary to corticosteroid increases during treatment [1]. When IOP is high, IOP should be lowered as soon as possible. This can be achieved by trying to reduce oral and topical steroids if the inflammation is controlled or treated with antiglaucoma drugs. Surgery should be performed if medical treatment is ineffective and intraocular pressure continues to rise [2]. Laser iridotomy appears to be less successful than surgical iridectomy in patients with angle closure secondary to pupillary block.

When filtering surgery is needed, supplementation with 5-fluorouracil or mitomycin C may increase the success rate of trabeculectomy. In patients with persistent inflammation, implantation drainage device may be the first choice [2].

14.3 Choroidal neovascularization and choroidal neovascular membrane

Choroidal neovascularization (CNV) is an important cause of late visual loss in patients with VKH. The presence of fundus pigmentation, chronic recurrent inflammation, and the recurrence of major anterior segment inflammation appear to be the risk factors for the development of CNV in VKH. CNV tends to develop in the peripapillary, subfoveal, and extrafoveal regions, where foci of inflammation seem to concentrate. Several treatment modalities including laser photocoagulation, photodynamic therapy, surgical excision, intravitreal steroid, and anti-vascular endothelial growth factor (anti-VEGF) therapy have been employed in the treatment of CNV secondary to VKH disease. Anti-VEGF injections have largely replaced PDT as the main treatment modality for CNV in recent years [1].

14.4 Subretinal fibrosis

Subretinal fibrosis is described in 8–40% of VKH cases, but is more common in chronic or recurrent cases. The most common locations are the peripapillary and extrafoveal regions. Histopathological findings show subretinal fibrosis, RPE cell metaplasia, and choroidal inflammatory cells. Fibrosis is induced when RPE cells, Müller cells, and choroidal fibroblasts interact with cytokines, immunoglobulins, and cellular mediators produced by T lymphocytes. The presence of subretinal fibrosis in VKH is associated with poor visual outcome [22].

15. Prognosis

VKH is a serious inflammatory disease, but prompt and aggressive treatment can lead to better visual outcomes. The use of corticosteroids and immunosuppressive agents has greatly improved the visual outcome in VKH patients [1]. Studies suggest final visual acuity can range from 20/20 to 20/50. Review of literature suggests starting treatment early and to treat with high-dose corticosteroids for at least 6 months. Treatment with steroid-sparing agents, including methotrexate, cyclosporine A, mycophenolate mofetil, or newer biologics, allows patients to use low-dose steroids while maintaining control of disease (**Figure 5**). The disease affects multiple organs, thus requiring coordination with other specialties, such as rheumatologist and neurologist. Several imaging modalities can be used to evaluate subclinical disease, including ICG angiography, fundus autofluorescence, and OCT. It can result in a longer treatment duration, but it results in fewer instances of sunset glow fundus and choroidal thinning [2].

Good initial visual acuity leads to better final visual outcomes, and initiating treatment in the acute phase yields more favorable outcomes than treating the disease in the chronic relapsing phase. Final visual outcome is better in eyes with fewer complications. Cataracts and glaucoma are the most common complications of VKH and can be treated surgically as long as the uveitis is controlled with medication. Perioperative management of uveitis is an essential key in VKH.

16. Future

16.1 Optical coherence tomography angiography (OCTA)

More recently, optical coherence tomography (OCTA) angiography has emerged as a useful non-invasive imaging technique that provides in-depth detailed reconstructions of the retinal-choroidal microvasculature using intraluminal blood flow as an intrinsic contrast [46].

OCTA was found to be a sensitive tool for detecting abnormalities such as dynamic changes in the choriocapillary layer, manifesting as multiple dark areas of choriocapillary loss, indicating the presence of "flow voids" in VKH [76]. OCTA has also recently been shown to be an effective tool for identifying changes at choriocapillary level in eyes with acute VKH disease and monitoring disease regression, relapse, and persistence in combination with clinical examination and other imaging modalities [76].

OCTA imaging can aid in diagnosis by identifying features of true choriocapillaris ischemia in eyes with acute VKH disease. Further research is needed to determine the role of OCTA in the management of VKH.

17. Conclusion

In conclusion, Vogt-Koyanagi-Harada disease is a severe bilateral granulomatous panuveitis manifesting as serous retinal detachment, disc hyperemia, and vitritis associated with headaches, nausea, meningeal irritation, alopecia, vitiligo, and hearing disability. The extraocular manifestations of the disease are variable, but early detection and treatment are essential key. SD-OCT, fundus fluorescein angiography, and B-scan ultrasonography are useful in diagnosing this disease. No previous history of trauma helps to distinguish it from sympathetic ophthalmia. The disease is thought to be caused by autoimmunity against the peptide tyrosinase produced by melanocytes, which is also responsible for the depigmentation in this disease. Initial treatment consists of high-dose corticosteroids, followed by steroid-sparing therapy and slow tapering long-term corticosteroids, with focus on controlling the inflammatory response to prevent sequelae like sunset glow fundus, cataract, glaucoma, and rarely choroidal neovascularization, which can limit ultimate visual potential [2]. The overall prognosis is fair, with substantial number of patients achieving a visual acuity of 20/40 or better with early and aggressive corticosteroid treatment.

Financial disclosure

The authors declare that they have no financial interests related to the work described in this chapter.

Abbreviations

SD-OCT	spectral-domain optical coherence tomography
ICGA	indocyanine green angiogram
FFA	fundus fluorescein angiogram
FAF	fundus autofluorescence

DOI: http://dx.doi.org/10.5772/intechopen.111594

Author details

Anubhav Goyal*, Vineet Shah, Giridhar Anantharaman and Mahesh Gopalakrishnan
Department of Vitreo-Retina, Giridhar Eye Institute, Cochin, Kerala, India

*Address all correspondence to: dranubhavgoyal@gmail.com

References

[1] Foster CS, Vitale AT. Diagnosis & Treatment of Uveitis. 2nd ed. New Delhi, India: Jaypee Brothers Medical; 2013

[2] O'Keefe GA, Rao NA. Vogt-Koyanagi-Harada disease. Survey of Ophthalmology. 2017 Jan-Feb;**62**(1):1-25. DOI: 10.1016/j.survophthal.2016.05.002

[3] Pattison EM. Uveomeningo encephalitic syndrome (Vogt-Koyanagi-Harada). Archives of Neurology. 1965; **12**(2):197-205

[4] Sleiman R, Kurban M, Succaria F, Abbas O. Poliosis circumscripta: Overview and underlying causes. Journal of the American Academy of Dermatology. 2013;**69**(4):625-633

[5] Tesavibul N. Vogt-Koyanagi-Harada Disease. In: Diagnosis and Treatment of Uveitis. Jaypee Brothers Medical Publishers (P) Ltd.; 2013. pp. 1013–1013

[6] Vogt A. Fruhzeitiges ergrauen der Zilien und bemerkungen uber den sogenannten plotzlichen eintritt dieser veranderung. Klinische Monatsblätter für Augenheilkunde. 1906;**4**:228-242

[7] Harada E. Beitrag zur klinischen kenntnis von michteitriger choroiditis (choroiditis diffusa acta). Acta Ophthalmologica Japan. 1926;**30**: 356-378

[8] Koyanagi Y. Dysakusis, alopecia und poliosis bei schwerer uveitis nicht traumatischen ursprungs. Klinische Monatsblätter für Augenheilkunde. 1929;**82**:194-211

[9] Babel J. Syndrome de Vogt-Koyanagi (Uveite bilaterale, poliosis, alopecie, vitiligo et dysacousie). Schweizerische Medizinische Wochenschrift. 1932;**44**: 1136-1140

[10] Bruno MG, Mcpherson SD Jr. Harada's disease. American Journal of Ophthalmology. 1949;**32**(4):513-522. DOI: 10.1016/0002-9394(49)90876-4

[11] Ohno S, Char DH, Kimura SJ, O'Connor GR. Vogt-Koyanagi-Harada syndrome. American Journal of Ophthalmology. 1977;**83**(5):735-740. DOI: 10.1016/0002-9394(77)90142-8

[12] Snyder DA, Tessler HH. Vogt-Koyanagi-Harada syndrome. American Journal of Ophthalmology. 1980;**90**(1): 69-75. DOI: 10.1016/s0002-9394(14) 75078-0

[13] Beniz J, Forster DJ, Lean JS, Smith RE, Rao NA. Variations in clinical features of the Vogt-Koyanagi-Harada syndrome. Retina. 1991;**11**(3):275-280. DOI: 10.1097/00006982-199111030-00001

[14] Tesavibul N, Sansanayuth W. Vogt-Koyanagi-Harada disease in Thai patients. Journal of the Medical Association of Thailand. 2005;**88**(Suppl 9):S26-S30

[15] Murakami S, Inaba Y, Mochizuki M, Nakajima A, Urayama A. A nationwide survey on the occurrence of Vogt-Koyanagi-Harada disease in Japan. Japanese Journal of Ophthalmology. 1994;**38**(2):208-213

[16] Nussenblatt RB. Clinical studies of Vogt-Koyanagi-Harada's disease at the National Eye Institute, NIH, USA. Japanese Journal of Ophthalmology. 1988;**32**(3):330-333

[17] Rubsamen PE, Gass JD. Vogt-Koyanagi-Harada syndrome. Clinical course, therapy, and long-term visual outcome. Archives of Ophthalmology. 1991;**109**(5):682-687. DOI: 10.1001/archopht.1991.01080050096037

[18] Sugiura S. Vogt-Koyanagi-Harada disease. Japanese Journal of Ophthalmology. 1978;**22**:9-35

[19] Al-Muammar AM, Al-Mudhaiyan TM, Al Otaibi M, Abdo A, Abu El-Asrar AM. Vogt-Koyanagi-Harada disease occurring during interferon-alpha and ribavirin therapy for chronic hepatitis C virus infection. International Ophthalmology. 2010;**30**(5):611-613. DOI: 10.1007/s10792-010-9357-0

[20] Moorthy RS, Inomata H, Rao NA. Vogt-Koyanagi-Harada syndrome. Survey of Ophthalmology. 1995;**39**(4):265-292. DOI: 10.1016/s0039-6257(05)80105-5

[21] Rathinam SR, Vijayalakshmi P, Namperumalsamy P. Vogt-Koyanagi-Harada syndrome in children. Ocular Immunology and Inflammation. 1998;**6**: 155-161

[22] Cunningham ET Jr, Demetrius R, Frieden IJ, Emery HM, Irvine AR, Good WV. Vogt-Koyanagi-Harada syndrome in a 4-year old child. American Journal of Ophthalmology. 1995;**120**(5):675-677. DOI: 10.1016/s0002-9394(14)72219-6

[23] Damico FM, Bezerra FT, Silva GC d, Gasparin F, Yamamoto JH. New insights into Vogt-Koyanagi-Harada disease. Arquivos Brasileiros de Oftalmologia. 2009;**72**(3):413-420. DOI: 10.1590/s0004-27492009000300028

[24] Norose K, Yano A. Melanoma specific Th1 cytotoxic T lymphocyte lines in Vogt-Koyanagi-Harada disease. The British Journal of Ophthalmology. 1996;**80**(11):1002-1008. DOI: 10.1136/bjo.80.11.1002

[25] Sugita S, Sagawa K, Mochizuki M, Shichijo S, Itoh K. Melanocyte lysis by cytotoxic T lymphocytes recognizing the MART-1 melanoma antigen in HLA-A2 patients with Vogt-Koyanagi-Harada disease. International Immunology. 1996;**8**(5):799-803. DOI: 10.1093/intimm/8.5.799

[26] Weisz JM, Holland GN, Roer LN, Park MS, Yuge AJ, Moorthy RS, et al. Association between Vogt-Koyanagi-Harada syndrome and HLA-DR1 and -DR4 in Hispanic patients living in southern California. Ophthalmology. 1995;**102**(7):1012-1015. DOI: 10.1016/s0161-6420(95)30920-7

[27] Arellanes-García L, Bautista N, Mora P, Ortega-Larrocea G, Burguet A, Gorodezky C. HLA-DR is strongly associated with Vogt-Koyanagi-Harada disease in Mexican Mestizo patients. Ocular Immunology and Inflammation. 1998;**6**(2):93-100. DOI: 10.1076/ocii.6.2.93.4049

[28] Patil YB, Garg R, Rajguru JP. VKH syndrome: A new perspective for healthcare professionals. Journal of Family Medicine and Primary Care. 2020;**9**(1):31-35

[29] Rao NA, Gupta A, Dustin L, Chee SP, Okada AA, Khairallah M, et al. Frequency of distinguishing clinical features in Vogt-Koyanagi-Harada disease. Ophthalmology. 2010;**117**(3): 591–9-599.e1. DOI: 10.1016/j.ophtha.2009.08.030

[30] Read RW, Holland GN, Rao NA. Revised diagnostic criteria for Vogt-Koyanagi-Harada disease: Report of an international committee on nomenclature. American Journal of Ophthalmology. 2001;**131**(5):647-652

[31] Murugan SB. Commentary: Appraisal of histopathological correlations I Vogt-Koyanagi-Harada uveitis. Indian Journal of Ophthalmology. 2019;**67**:1219-1221

[32] Rao NA. Pathology of Vogt-Koyanagi-Harada disease. International Ophthalmology. 2007;**27**(2–3):81-85. DOI: 10.1007/s10792-006-9029-2

[33] Lavezzo MM, Sakata VM, Morita C, Rodriguez EE, Abdallah SF, Da Silva FT. Koyanagi-Harada disease: Review of rare autoimmune disease targeting antigens of melanocytes. Orphanet Journal of Rare Diseases. 2016 Mar;**24**:11:29. DOI: 10.1186/s13023-016-0412-4

[34] Das D, Boddepalli A, Biswas J. Clinicopathological and immuno histochemistry correlation in a case of Vogt-Koyanagi-Harada disease. Indian Journal of Ophthalmology. 2019;**67**(7): 1217-1219. DOI: 10.4103/ijo.IJO_1800_18

[35] Lavezzo MM, Sakata VM, Morita C, Rodriguez EEC, Abdallah SF, da Silva FTG, et al. Vogt-Koyanagi-Harada disease: Review of a rare autoimmune disease targeting antigens of melanocytes. Orphanet Journal of Rare Diseases. 2016;**11**(1):29. DOI: 10.1186/s13023-016-0412-4

[36] Kato Y, Kurimura M, Yahata Y, Tajima K, Kato T. Vogt-Koyanagi-Harada's disease presenting polymorphonuclear pleocytosis in the cerebrospinal fluid at the early active stage. Internal Medicine. 2006;**45**(12):779-781. DOI: 10.2169/internalmedicine.45.1669

[37] Lubin JR, Loewenstein JI, Frederick AR Jr. Vogt-Koyanagi-Harada syndrome with focal neurologic signs. American Journal of Ophthalmology. 1981;**91**(3): 332-341. DOI: 10.1016/0002-9394(81)90286-5

[38] Trebini F, Appiotti A, Bacci R, Daniele D, Inglezis A, Scarzella G. Vogt-Koyanagi-Harada syndrome: Clinical and instrumental contribution. Italian Journal of Neurological Sciences. 1991; **12**(5):479-484

[39] Minakawa R, Ohno S, Hirose S. Clinical manifestations of Vogt-Koyanagi-Harada disease. Japanese Journal of Ophthalmology. 1988;**39**:1249-1253

[40] Hoshi H, Tamada Y, Murata Y. Changes in audiogram in the course of Harada's disease. Japanese Journal of Ophthalmology. 1977;**31**:23-30

[41] Usui Y, Goto H, Sakai J-I, Takeuchi M, Usui M, Rao NA. Presumed Vogt-Koyanagi-Harada disease with unilateral ocular involvement: report of three cases. Arbeitsphysiologie. 2009; **247**(8):1127-1132. DOI: 10.1007/s00417-009-1068-8

[42] Neves A, Cardoso A, Almeida M, Campos J, Campos A, Castro Sousa JP. Unilateral Vogt-Koyanagi-Harada disease: A clinical case report. Case Reports in Ophthalmology. 2015;**6**(3): 361-365. DOI: 10.1159/000441616

[43] Cunningham ET Jr, Rathinam SR, Tugal-Tutkun I, Muccioli C, Zierhut M. Vogt-Koyanagi-Harada disease. Ocular Immunology and Inflammation. 2014; **22**(4):249-252. DOI: 10.3109/09273948.2014.939530

[44] Forster DJ, Green RL, Rao NA. Unilateral manifestation of the Vogt-Koyanagi-Harada syndrome in a 7-year-old child. American Journal of Ophthalmology. 1991;**111**(3):380-382. DOI: 10.1016/s0002-9394(14)72334-7

[45] Da Silva FT, Hirata CE, Olivalves E, Oyamada MK, Yamamoto JH. Fundus-based and electroretinographic strategies for stratification of late-stage Vogt-Koyanagi-Harada disease patients. American Journal of Ophthalmology. 2009;**148**(6):939-945

[46] Agrawal R, Xin W, Keane PA, Chhablani J, Agarwal A. Optical

coherence tomography angiography: A non-invasive tool to image end-arterial system. Expert Review of Medical Devices. 2016;**13**(6):519-521. DOI: 10.1080/17434440.2016.1186540

[47] Sakata VM, da Silva FT, Hirata CE, de Carvalho JF, Yamamoto JH. Diagnosis and classification of Vogt-Koyanagi-Harada disease. Autoimmunity Reviews. 2014;**13**(4–5):550-555. DOI: 10.1016/j.autrev.2014.01.023

[48] Fardeau C, Tran TH, Gharbi B, Cassoux N, Bodaghi B, Lehoang P. Of 21 tomography in successive stages of Vogt-Koyanagi-Harada disease. Orphanet Journal of Rare Diseases. 2007;**11**(2–3): 163-172

[49] Arellanes-Garcia L, Hernandez-Barrios M, Fromow-Guerra J, Cervantes-FP. Fluorescein fundus angiographic findings in Vogt-Koyanagi- Harada syndrome. International Ophthalmology. 2007;**27**(2–3):155-161

[50] Stanga PE, Lim JI, Hamilton P. Indocyanine green angiography in chorioretinal diseases: Indications and interpretation: An evidence-based update. Ophthalmology. 2003;**110**(1): 15-21. DOI: 10.1016/s0161-6420(02)01563-4

[51] Herbort CP, LeHoang P, Guex-Crosier Y. Schematic interpretation of indocyanine green angiography in posterior uveitis using a standard angiographic protocol. Ophthalmology. 1998;**105**(3):432-440. DOI: 10.1016/S0161-6420(98)93024-X

[52] Herbort CP, Mantovani A, Bouchenaki N. Indocyanine green angiography in Vogt-Koyanagi-Harada disease: Angiographic signs and utility in patient follow-up. International Ophthalmology. 2007;**27**(2–3):173-182. DOI: 10.1007/s10792-007-9060-y

[53] Koizumi H, Maruyama K, Kinoshita S. Blue light and near-infrared fundus autofluorescence in acute Vogt-Koyanagi-Harada disease. The British Journal of Ophthalmology. 2010;**94**(11): 1499-1505. DOI: 10.1136/bjo.2009.164665

[54] Heussen FM, Vasconcelos-Santos DV, Pappuru RR, Walsh AC, Rao NA, Sadda SR. Ultra-wide-field green-light (532-nm) autofluorescence imaging in chronic Vogt-Koyanagi-Harada disease. Ophthalmic Surgery, Lasers & Imaging. 2011;**42**(4):272-277. DOI: 10.3928/15428877-20110505-01

[55] Ishihara K, Hangai M, Kita M, Yoshimura N. Acute Vogt-Koyanagi-Harada disease in enhanced spectral-domain optical coherence tomography. Ophthalmology. 2009;**116**(9):1799-1807. DOI: 10.1016/j.ophtha.2009.04.002

[56] Nazari H, Rao NA. Resolution of subretinal fluid with systemic corticosteroid treatment in acute Vogt-Koyanagi-Harada disease. The British Journal of Ophthalmology. 2012;**96**(11): 1410-1414. DOI: 10.1136/bjophthalmol-2012-301857

[57] Zhao C, Zhang M-F, Dong F-T, Wang X-Q, Wen X, Dai R-P, et al. Spectral domain optical coherence tomography of Vogt-Koyanagi-Harada disease: Novel findings and new insights into the pathogenesis. Chinese Medical Sciences Journal. 2012;**27**(1): 29-34. DOI: 10.1016/s1001-9294(12)60019-4

[58] Vasconcelos-Santos DV, Sohn EH, Sadda S, Rao NA. Retinal pigment epithelial changes in chronic Vogt-Koyanagi-Harada disease: Fundus autofluorescence and spectral domain-optical coherence tomography findings. Retina. 2010;**30**(1):33-41. DOI: 10.1097/IAE.0b013e3181c5970d

[59] Hashizume K, Imamura Y, Fujiwara T, Machida S, Ishida M, Kurosaka D. Choroidal thickness in eyes with posterior recurrence of Vogt-Koyanagi-Harada disease after high-dose steroid therapy. Acta Ophthalmologica. 2014;**92**(6):e490-e491

[60] da Silva FT, Sakata VM, Nakashima A, Hirata CE, Olivalves E, Takahashi WY, et al. Enhanced depth imaging optical coherence tomography in long-standing Vogt-Koyanagi-Harada disease. The British Journal of Ophthalmology. 2013;**97**(1):70-74. DOI: 10.1136/bjophthalmol-2012-302089

[61] Forster DJ, Cano MR, Green RL, Rao NA. Echographic features of the Vogt- Koyanagi-Harada syndrome. Archives of Ophthalmology. 1990; **108**(10):1421-1426

[62] Gohdo T, Tsukahara S. Ultrasound Biomicroscopy of shallow anterior chamber in Vogt-Koyanagi-Harada syndrome. American Journal of Ophthalmology. 1996;**122**(1): 112-114. DOI: 10.1016/s0002-9394(14) 71973-7

[63] Chee SP, Luu CD, Cheng CL, Lim WK, Jap A. Visual function in Vogt-Koyanagi-Harada patients. Graefe's Archive for Clinical and Experimental Ophthalmology. 2005;**243**(8):785-790

[64] Yang P, Fang W, Wang L, Wen F, Wu W, Kijlstra A. Study of macular function by multifocal electroretinography in patients with Vogt-Koyanagi-Harada syndrome. American Journal of Ophthalmology. 2008;**146**(5):767-771. DOI: 10.1016/j. ajo.2008.05.044

[65] Rishi P, Appanraj R, Sharma T. Choroidal melanoma masquerading as multifocal central serous chorioretinopathy. Oman Journal of Ophthalmology. 2016;**9**(3):187-188. DOI: 10.4103/0974-620X.192305

[66] Ushio R, Yamamoto M, Miyasaka A, Muraoka T, Kanaoka H, Tamura H, et al. Nivolumab-induced Vogt-Koyanagi-Harada-like syndrome and adrenocortical insufficiency with long-term survival in a patient with non-small-cell lung cancer. Internal Medicine. 2021;**60**(22):3593-3598. DOI: 10.2169/internalmedicine.6410-20

[67] Gambichler T, Seifert C, Lehmann M, Lukas C, Scheel C, Susok L. Concurrent Vogt-Koyanagi-Harada disease and impressive response to immune checkpoint blockade in metastatic melanoma. Immunotherapy. 2020;**12**(7): 439-444. DOI: 10.2217/imt-2019-0206

[68] Diamantopoulos PT, Stoungioti S, Anastasopoulou A, Papaxoinis G, Gogas H. Incomplete Vogt-Koyanagi-Harada disease following treatment with encorafenib and binimetinib for metastatic melanoma. Melanoma Research. 2018; **28**(6):648-651. DOI: 10.1097/ CMR.0000000000000505

[69] Williams BK Jr, Di Nicola M, Lucio-Alvarez JA, Lally DR, Shields CL. Choroidal melanoma simulating adenoma of the retinal pigment epithelium arising at the site of congenital hypertrophy of the retinal pigment epithelium. Ocular Oncology and Pathology. 2020;**6**(1):39-43. DOI: 10.1159/000501084

[70] Iwata D, Mizuuchi K, Aoki K, Horie Y, Kase S, Namba K, et al. Serial frequencies and clinical features of uveitis in Hokkaido, Japan. Ocular Immunology and Inflammation. 2017;**25** (sup1):S15-S18. DOI: 10.1080/ 09273948.2016.1184286

[71] Fernandez G, Nascimento D, Nascimento H, Muccioli C, Belfort C.

Uveitis in São Paulo, Brazil: 1053 New Patients in 15 months. Ocular Immunology and Inflammation. 2017; **25**(3):382-387

[72] Trancoso FG, Gallon L, Bomfim ML d A, AFM da S, Cade F, Zanetti FR. Optical coherence tomography angiography findings in patients with Alport syndrome. Arquivos Brasileiros de Oftalmologia. 2020;**83**(6):473-477. DOI: 10.5935/0004-2749.20200088

[73] Bhandari GS, Duggal L, Jain N, Patel J. Cogan syndrome: An autoimmune eye and ear disease with systemic manifestations. National Medical Journal of India. 2019;**32**(6): 349-351. DOI: 10.4103/ 0970-258X.303611

[74] Dammacco R, Biswas J, Kivelä TT, Zito FA, Leone P, Mavilio A, et al. Ocular sarcoidosis: Clinical experience and recent pathogenetic and therapeutic advancements. International Ophthalmology. 2020;**40**(12):3453-3467. DOI: 10.1007/s10792-020-01531-0

[75] Ghem MRD, Hungaro AC, Hokazono K. Serous retinal detachment as an Early manifestation of lúpus choroidopathy. Arquivos Brasileiros de Oftalmologia. 2021;**84**(6):594-597. DOI: 10.5935/0004-2749.20210097

[76] Aggarwal K, Agarwal A, Mahajan S, Invernizzi A, Mandadi SKR, Singh R, et al. The role of optical coherence tomography angiography in the diagnosis and management of acute Vogt-Koyanagi-Harada disease. Ocular Immunology and Inflammation. 2018; **26**(1):142-153. DOI: 10.1080/ 09273948.2016.1195001

Chapter 5

Malignancies Masquerading as Uveitis

Teresa E. Fowler and Diego Espinosa-Heidmann

Abstract

Malignancy presenting as uveitis can be symptomatically mild and difficult to diagnose, often leading to delayed treatment and poor outcomes. In this chapter, we describe the range of malignancies reported to present with uveitis, both primary ocular malignancies and systemic malignancies which metastasize to the eye. We describe the range of clinical features and corresponding complaints that may be encountered with specific malignancies and provide a thorough review of diagnostic tools available to aid in diagnosis. The primary goal of this chapter is to aid in the diagnosis of intraocular malignancy to reduce treatment delays and improve patient outcomes.

Keywords: malignancy, uveitis, intraocular malignancy, metastatic ocular disease, lymphoma, leukemia, uveal melanoma

1. Introduction

The presence of intraocular cell does not always imply a primary inflammatory condition. It is reported that approximately 5% of patients initially diagnosed with uveitis have an underlying masquerade syndrome, about half of which are from a malignant process [1]. Intraocular cells in these cases may be inflammatory cells released in response to a separate primary condition or maybe entirely unrelated entities, such as heme, pigment, or malignant cells easily mistaken for inflammatory cells.

Although ocular immune privilege generally protects the eye from immune attack, malignant intraocular lesions may directly or indirectly incite an inflammatory response. Direct expression of antigenic proteins by a cancerous lesion can cause secondary uveitis [2, 3], with typical symptoms including redness, pain, photophobia, and blurred vision. Hematologic malignancies invading the eye may cause anterior chamber cell, vitritis, or retinochoroiditis clinically indistinguishable from an inflammatory uveitis flare. Malignancies manifesting as intraocular cells are important to keep on the differential but can present a diagnostic challenge, as their subjective and objective features can be nearly identical to the inflammatory uveitis triggered by infectious or noninfectious causes. Additionally, haze in the anterior or posterior chambers can impede the complete evaluation of the eye.

Malignancies are among the most feared uveitis masquerade syndromes, as delay in diagnosis and treatment can result in fatality. Clinical judgment and thorough evaluation are paramount in arriving at the correct diagnosis; intraocular malignancies often come to light when an astute provider notes uveitis features with a negative workup and treatment failure with anti-inflammatory medications, pursuing further workup as detailed below.

1.1 Diagnostic tools

The provider caring for a patient with presumed uveitis who is not responding to anti-inflammatory treatments as expected has several diagnostic tools available for further investigation, some of which may be readily available in the office. A thorough ophthalmic exam is critical, with detailed documentation of the affected ocular segments. Since intraocular biopsy is invasive and poses a risk of vision-threatening complications, much of the diagnostic support for a diagnosis of intraocular malignancy relies on noninvasive testing.

1.1.1 Noninvasive or minimally invasive in-office testing

Fundus photography is helpful for monitoring the evolution of disease over time, as well as treatment response. These images can be used to document lesion dimensions, pigmentation, presence of drusen or lipofuscin, lacunae, vascular abnormalities, infarcts, and retinal atrophy. Fundus photography may also be helpful in patients with difficulty cooperating with the slit lamp and indirect examination. When a diagnosis of malignancy is uncertain, fundus photography provides a detailed snapshot that, in combination with a detailed clinical examination, can be monitored over time.

Optical coherence tomography (OCT) utilizes the reflection and scattering of light waves to create high-resolution cross-sectional imaging of the retinal layers [4]. OCT images have higher sensitivity for detecting retinal edema, thinning, atrophy, and subretinal fluid than clinical examination alone [5]. For some ocular malignancies, features such as subretinal fluid or nodularity have been shown to be associated with risk for metastasis, so OCT can be particularly helpful in understanding the full spectrum of disease in these patients [6]. OCT of the optic nerve can be helpful in monitoring nerve edema or atrophy. In cases with dense vitreous haze or a poor view of the posterior segment, OCT is of limited use and alternative testing methods must be employed. OCT is widely available, rapid, relatively inexpensive, and technically straightforward to perform, making it one of the best initial tests for understanding complex ophthalmic disease.

Additional widely available noninvasive imaging includes fundus autofluorescence (FAF), a modality based on the differential absorption of specific wavelengths of light by ocular tissues. Lesions can be described as hyper- or hypo-autofluorescent based on their appearance. Hyperautofluorescence, seen as light coloration, indicates the presence of fluorophores excited by blue or green light and emitting light of longer wavelengths. Lipofuscin and related compounds are readily autofluorescent; thus, healthy RPE appears light on FA. Normal hypo-autofluorescent tissues include the vasculature since heme strongly absorbs blue and green wavelengths without excitation, and the optic nerve, which does not contain RPE or lipofuscin fluorophores. RPE and lipofuscin accumulation, as seen in choroidal melanomas and metastatic lesions, causes hyperautofluorescence, whereas nevi and congenital RPE hypertrophy appear hypo-autofluorescent. Areas of RPE atrophy appear dark and are referred to as "window defects."

Ultrasound biomicroscopy, a technique using high-frequency sound waves to look at the anterior segment, and B-scan ultrasound, using lower-frequency sound with a greater depth of focus, are noninvasive and can provide valuable clues to the underlying diagnosis. Biomicroscopy is particularly useful for lesions in the angle or far peripheral retina, where they may be difficult to view with a slit lamp or indirect exam. B-scan can be used to evaluate and measure posterior segment lesions, as well as for surgical planning, especially when the view is limited by vitreous haze or anterior segment pathology. The acoustic properties of the lesion are helpful in diagnosis; for example, choroidal melanoma likely has a dome or mushroom shape with moderate reflectivity, whereas retinoblastoma contains hyperreflective calcium deposits [7].

1.1.2 Evaluation for metastasis

In patients with suspected or confirmed malignancy, computed tomography (CT) and magnetic resonance imaging (MRI) imaging of sites suspected to be involved, including the CNS, are critical in evaluating for metastasis. Cerebrospinal fluid analysis via lumbar puncture with cytology and cytokine analysis can identify malignant cells unable to be seen on imaging. Suspicious brain lesions may require biopsy. The presence of intracranial or intrathecal lesions significantly changes both management and prognosis. Additional imaging may be indicated depending on the diagnosis.

1.1.3 Invasive testing and cytologic studies

For some intraocular malignancies, diagnostic vitrectomy or vitreous aspiration is the only means of a definitive diagnosis. Of course, either technique carries the risk of devastating complications leading to vision loss or loss of the eye and, in some cases, the risk of seeding the malignancy, so this decision should be carefully considered. Since the vitreous is relatively acellular, malignant cells can be scattered, and false negative results are possible. Malignant cells are especially sensitive to changing conditions, so samples must be delicately handled and rapidly processed. Careful fine-needle aspiration of retinal or choroidal tumors may be performed concurrently or at a later time for a more condensed sample of cells if vitrectomy is nondiagnostic [8].

Once the sample is obtained, it is processed through several testing techniques for diagnosis. Cytologic studies can differentiate inflammatory cells from malignant ones based on characteristic features. Malignant cells tend to be large with abnormally segmented nuclei, scant cytoplasm, and abundant nucleoli [9, 10]. Benign inflammatory cells, on the other hand, are smaller, with characteristic nuclear and cytoplasmic features based on cell type. The presence of necrotic cells is suggestive of malignancy, as these are not typically present in an uveitic reaction.

Immunophenotyping, a method for identifying cells based on expressed surface markers, can be used to differentiate cell populations. Malignancies arise from the uncontrolled proliferation of homogenous cell populations, which can be identified based on markers, such as CD19, CD20, and CD22 on the surface of B cells. Flow cytometry can sort cells based on the presence of several markers and may be diagnostic even when cytology is inconclusive [1]. The diagnosis can also be supported by polymerase chain reaction (PCR), a technique used to identify specific gene mutations or rearrangements present in sample tissue [11].

Cytokine analysis can be particularly helpful in differentiating inflammatory uveitis from malignancy. Interleukin (IL) cytokines are immune-modulating proteins secreted by inflammatory cells with a host of functions. For example, IL-6 is a pro-inflammatory signal secreted by B and T cells, whereas IL-10 is an inflammatory inhibitor produced by T helper cells. Specific cytokines may be released from malignant cells, so the cytokine profile of a sample identified by enzyme-linked immunosorbent assay (ELISA) can aid in diagnosis.

2. Hematologic malignancies masquerading as uveitis

2.1 Leukemia

Leukemic cancers arise from bone marrow-derived blood cells. Acute leukemia and blast crises can rarely present with uveitis findings. Reported clinical findings range from low-grade anterior chamber cells to dense pseudohypopyon with intermixed heme [12]. Vitreous cell is less common in chronic leukemia but may be present in an acute blast crisis, and may be indicative of CNS involvement [13]. Anti-inflammatory agents are ineffective in treatment. Anterior chamber aspirate may reveal leukemic cells, with or without blast cells [13]. Patients with a known diagnosis of leukemia in remission should be evaluated for relapse when presenting with uveitic findings [13]. Intraocular findings more common in leukemia include retinal hemorrhages in all layers, often with white centers indicative of capillary rupture or leukemic cell aggregation.

2.2 Lymphoid malignancies

Lymphomas comprise a group of malignancies arising from B or T lymphocytes. Lymphoid malignancies occurring within the eye may be differentiated into vitreoretinal or uveal based on their origins. Systemic lymphoma spread hematogenously to the eye may present with visual decline, floaters, photophobia, or eye pain. The spectrum of clinical features similar to uveitis may include pseudohypopyon, anterior chamber cells, vitritis, white subretinal infiltrates, vascular inflammation, or choroiditis. Choroidal masses or whitening may be the primary feature. These malignant proliferations of B or T cells can easily be mistaken for inflammatory uveitis, and delays in an accurate diagnosis can lead to poor outcomes.

3. Central nervous system malignancies

3.1 Primary vitreoretinal lymphoma (PVRL)

The most common intraocular lymphoid malignancy, and one frequently misdiagnosed as uveitis, is PVRL. The vast majority of PVRL is non-Hodgkin B cell lymphomas [14], primarily involving the CNS, whereas rare cases arise from T cells [15]. The incidence of PVRL peaks in the 6th and 7th decades of life [16], with immunocompromised individuals being at higher risk than the general public. Human immunodeficiency virus (HIV) with a low CD-4 count is a known risk factor, so clinicians diagnosing uveitis in a known HIV-positive or otherwise immunocompromised patient should have PVRL on the differential [17]. PVRL is often initially misdiagnosed, with patients being treated for alternative conditions for 10–21 months and undergoing four or more diagnostic procedures before the correct diagnosis is made [1, 10].

3.1.1 PVRL presentation and clinical features

Presenting complaints and clinical features vary. Two-thirds of patients have bilateral involvement [18], though findings can be highly asymmetric. Visual haze, blurriness, and floaters are common complaints [18]. Cells within the anterior segment may range from scarce to dense, sometimes evolving into a layered pseudo-hypopyon [19]. Patients generally do not develop posterior synechiae. In the posterior segment, vitritis with large, homogenous cells and lymphocyte clumping is often present. A heavy lymphocyte burden in the trabecular meshwork can lead to secondary glaucoma [16].

An important clinical finding suggestive of PRVL, though found in only one in five patients, is the presence of creamy yellow subretinal infiltrates composed of accumulated malignant lymphocytes beneath the RPE [20], which appear hyper-reflective on OCT and hyperautofluorescent on FAF. These subretinal infiltrates can shift over time and may lead to areas of geographic atrophy. Subretinal fluid may be seen over infiltrates. Accumulation of atypical lymphocytes along vasculature can compromise perfusion and lead to ischemia, with downstream neovascular consequences. Involvement of the optic disc may be seen clinically as optic nerve head edema and elevation.

The symptoms of PVRL are often mild and insidious, leading to delayed presentation. It is estimated that symptoms are present for an average of 6 months before diagnosis, though patients treated for chronic smoldering uveitis for 2 years or more prior to PVRL diagnosis have been reported. Patients may temporarily improve with topical or systemic steroids, but later recur.

3.1.2 PVRL diagnosis and treatment

Workup often begins with negative blood work and chest x-ray to rule out causes of inflammatory uveitis. Office-based testing may include OCT, demonstrating subretinal infiltrates or subretinal fluid, FAF with hyperautofluorescent subretinal lesions, or fluorescein angiogram (FA) with hyperfluorescent lesions and window defects [21]. Hypocyanescence on indocyanine green angiography can be helpful in distinguishing PVRL from white dot syndromes [22].

When PVRL is suspected, vitrectomy is performed to obtain vitreous samples and may be accompanied by a subretinal aspiration biopsy of selected lesions [23]. Cytology reveals a mix of typical inflammatory cells with malignant lymphocytes, distinguishable by their large size, atypical nuclei, scarce cytoplasm, and numerous nucleoli. Intermixed necrotic cells are not typical of inflammatory uveitis and, therefore, support the diagnosis of malignancy.

Immunohistochemical staining can be used to demonstrate B-cell-specific markers, such as CD19, CD20, CD22, and Pax-5 [24]. MYD88, a protein encoded on chromosome 3 with immune signaling functions, is found to be mutated in up to 70% of PVRL [25]. The ratio of interleukin 10 (IL-10), an anti-inflammatory cytokine, to IL-6, its pro-inflammatory counterpart, suggests malignancy when greater than 1 or benign inflammation when less than 1. Monoclonality on gene rearrangement studies is a feature of malignancy, as well as the predominance of a specific light chain subtype. Even with all of these testing methods, false negatives are unfortunately common due to the paucicellular composition of vitreous, delicate tissue processing, and small sample sizes [10].

All patients undergoing workup for PVRL should undergo neuroimaging and cerebrospinal fluid analysis to evaluate for CNS involvement. CNS involvement is common, seen in up to 2/3 of PVRL patients [21], and confers a poor prognosis. Treatment involves intravitreal chemotherapy, generally with serial methotrexate [26, 27] and/or rituximab [28], and ocular radiation. Response to treatment may be monitored in the office using the imaging techniques described above [22]. Patients with CNS lesions require systemic or intrathecal chemotherapy, as well as extensive radiation. Despite aggressive treatment, the prognosis remains poor [21].

4. Non-hematologic malignancies masquerading as uveitis

4.1 Metastases from distant primary cancers

The vascularity of the choroid makes it a common area for metastatic invasion. Blurred vision in a patient with a recent or distant history of cancer, especially breast or lung cancer [29], should raise suspicion. Approximately 1/3 of patients diagnosed with a choroidal metastatic lesion do not have a known diagnosis of cancer prior to their presentation for eye complaints [29]. Clinical features include a unilateral dome-shaped choroidal elevation without significant pigmentation, with adjacent shifting subretinal fluid, which may require OCT for diagnosis. B-scan may demonstrate an echogenic lesion within the choroid, with or without overlying subretinal fluid or detachment (**Figures 1** and **2**).

4.2 Uveal melanoma

Melanoma of the uvea is the most frequently diagnosed primary ocular malignancy [30–33] and comprises approximately 5% of melanomas [34]. The prognosis is strongly correlated with the size of the primary tumor at diagnosis [35]; thus, prompt and accurate diagnosis is crucial as delay may be fatal. Uveal melanoma is most commonly observed in Caucasian [36] patients in their 6th to 7th decade of life [34, 37]. Symptomatic patients may complain of blurred vision, photopsias, or visual field defects, though a significant proportion is asymptomatic and identified on routine screening exams [31].

Small choroidal melanomas may be overlooked on early examinations or may be obscured from clinical views by the iris. Anterior or posterior chamber cells may be the first indication of a choroidal melanoma; in these cases, the intraocular cells are composed of inflammatory cells, pigment cells, and malignant cells [38]. In a pig model, inflammatory uveitis thought to be the result of an immunologic cross-reaction has been shown to develop in response to cutaneous melanoma [39], suggesting a potential mechanism for intraocular cells. Epithelioid cell-predominant melanomas have been shown to cause more inflammation than spindle or type A melanoma cells [40].

Clinical examination of uveal melanoma typically reveals a unilaterally elevated subretinal lesion with brown or gray coloration. If penetration through the Bruch membrane occurs, the tumor may extend into the vitreous via a stalk through the retina, taking on a “mushroom” shape. If the lesion is sharply defined or overlying drusen are present, a benign nevus or hypertrophy of the RPE should be considered.

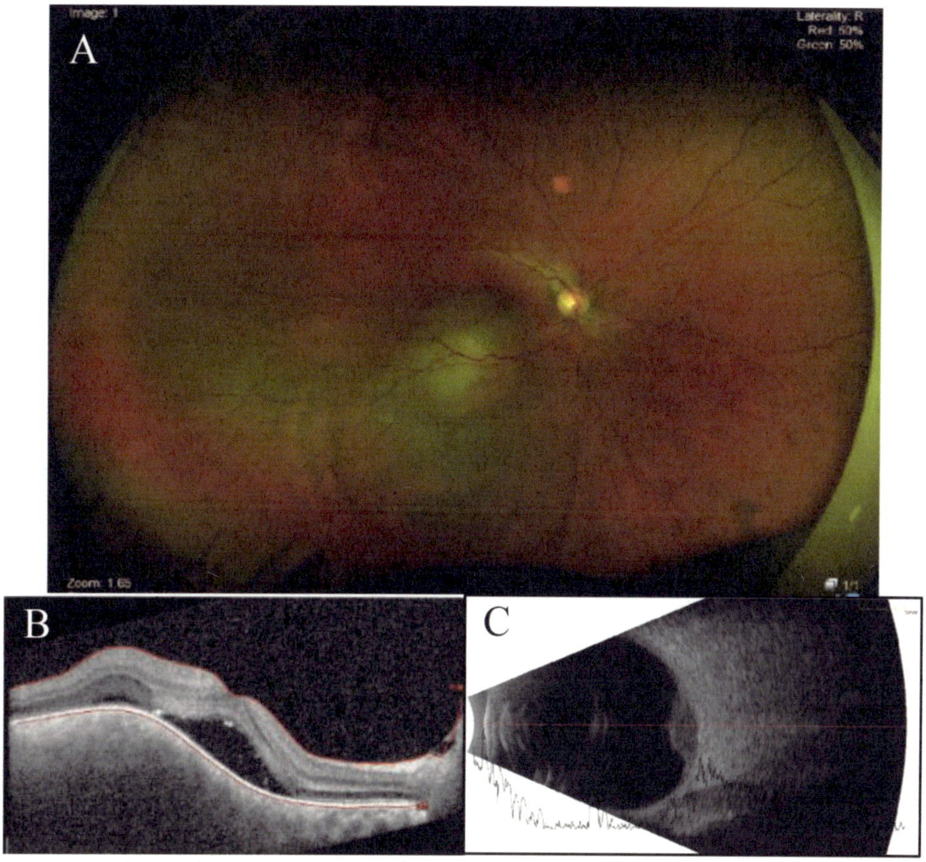

Figure 1.
Choroidal metastasis with exudative macular detachment from Ewing sarcoma. A patient with a known history of Ewing sarcoma undergoing systemic therapy presented with complaints of decreased visual acuity with constant distortion and intermittent flashes in the right eye (OD). (A) Fundus photograph of the right eye showing a choroidal mass within the inferior macula. (B) OCT of the right macula showing a fovea-involving exudative retinal detachment overlying the choroidal mass. (C) B-scan ultrasonography of the same patient demonstrating a choroidal mass lesion with medium reflectivity measuring 9.6 × 11 mm at its base and 3.5 mm in height. Images courtesy of Dr. Diego Espinosa-Heidmann.

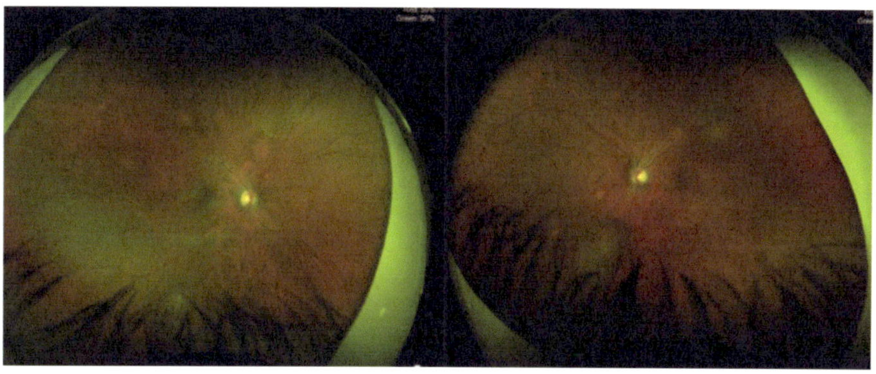

Figure 2.
Multifocal choroidal metastases from a primary neuroendocrine malignancy. Fundus photograph showing multiple orange-yellow choroidal lesions of varying sizes in the mid-periphery bilaterally. In this case, the primary malignancy was a high-grade neuroendocrine tumor identified in the lung. Image courtesy of Dr. Diego Espinosa-Heidmann.

Features suggestive of melanoma include thickness greater than 2 mm, subretinal fluid, orange lipofuscin, dilated or tortuous overlying vasculature, and close proximity to the optic nerve.

Ultrasound of a uveal melanoma demonstrates low to medium internal echogenicity with orbital shadowing beyond the lesion [41] and can be used to measure tumor dimensions and assess for orbital invasion. Ultrasound biomicroscopy may provide a better assessment of ciliary body tumors. Fluorescein angiography may show vessel irregularity or leakage around the tumor, as well as the classic "double circulation" sign with retinal and tumor vessels simultaneously visible [42]. A fine-needle aspiration biopsy provides a definitive histopathological diagnosis [43]. Melanoma has the propensity to spread hematogenously, with metastatic spread observed in up to 50% [44], and increasing tumor thickness has been shown to correlate with a higher risk of metastasis [6]. Once a primary tumor is identified, evaluation for the metastatic disease should proceed with imaging of the central nervous system, liver, and lungs. Prognosis strongly correlates with tumor size; survival is greater than 80% for tumors less than 10 mm but only approximately 40% for those with diameters greater than 16 mm [45].

Treatment of uveal melanoma historically included enucleation and localized radiotherapy until the mid-1970s, though there was concern that enucleation facilitated metastatic dissemination [46, 47]. The Collaborative Ocular Melanoma Study (COMS), a prospective multicenter randomized trial comparing treatment outcomes for uveal melanoma, began in 1985 and followed enrolled patients until 2003. The main conclusions from COMS include (1) equal 5-year survival for medium uveal melanoma patients treated with brachytherapy versus enucleation [48] and (2) no improvement in outcomes for large melanomas treated with radiation prior to enucleation compared to enucleation alone [49, 50]. Localized proton beam radiotherapy using externally applied protons, carbon, or helium particles has also shown promise in the treatment of large melanomas [51] (**Figure 3**).

4.3 Retinoblastoma

Retinoblastoma is a childhood cancer of neuroendocrine origin, the most recognized manifestation of which is leukocoria. An estimated 50% of patients referred to ocular oncologists with concern for retinoblastoma end up having alternate diagnoses [52]. In up to 3% of retinoblastoma patients, intraocular cell may be the presenting finding [53, 54], especially for the diffuse infiltrating subtype. Retinoblastoma should be on the differential for young patients presenting with signs and symptoms of uveitis without a clear underlying etiology (**Figure 4**).

4.3.1 Diffuse infiltrating retinoblastoma

Diffuse infiltrating retinoblastoma is a rare subtype of retinoblastoma known to mimic uveitis. Of the 7000–8000 retinoblastoma cases diagnosed annually [55], approximately 2% are diffuse infiltrating [54]. Rather than form a distinct mass, as in typical retinoblastoma, malignant cells in this subtype spread tangentially along and within the retina in an ill-defined and irregular pattern, with the tumor seeding throughout the eye. Suggested mechanisms behind this atypical growth pattern include immune dysregulation [56] or mutations of cell adhesion molecules [57], though strong evidence is lacking.

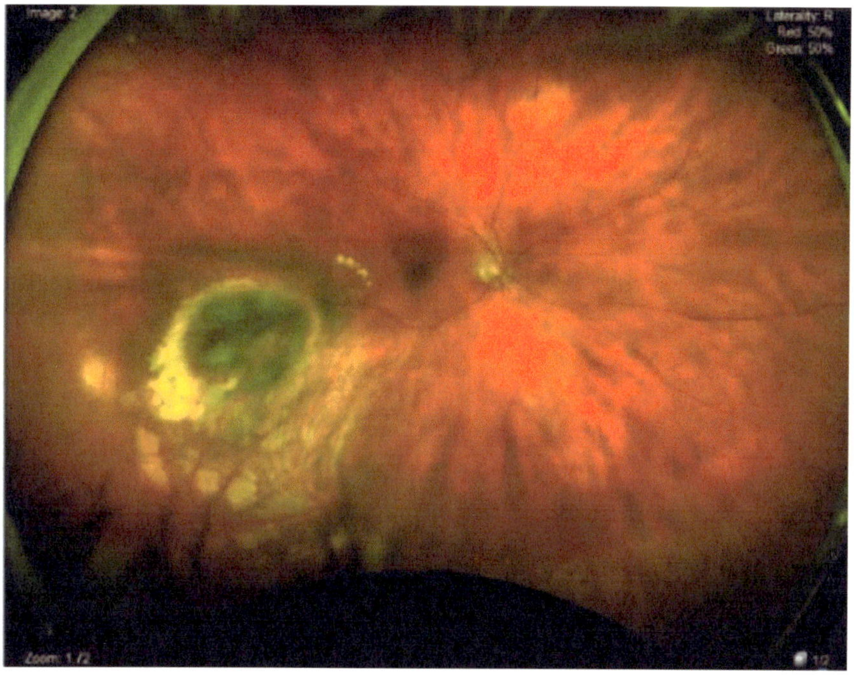

Figure 3.
Choroidal melanoma status post brachytherapy and thermotherapy. Fundus photograph of the right eye demonstrating an irregularly pigmented inferotemporal lesion with surrounding retinal atrophy consistent with a regressed choroidal melanoma. This lesion was closely monitored for recurrence. Image courtesy of Dr. Espinosa-Heidmann.

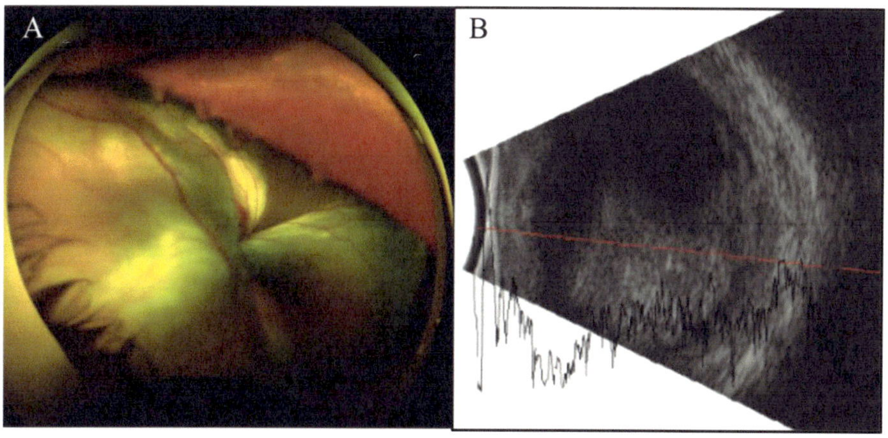

Figure 4.
Retinoblastoma in a 3-year-old child referred by a pediatrician due to leukocoria of the right eye. Family history included retinoblastoma requiring enucleation in an older sibling. (A) Fundus photograph showing a yellow-white mass in the posterior pole with associated exudative detachment, and (B) B-scan ultrasonography of the same eye demonstrating a large macula-involving elevated intraocular mass with high internal reflectivity. Images courtesy of Dr. Espinosa-Heidmann.

Much of our knowledge of this relatively rare disease comes from published case reports and series. The average age of presentation for this subtype is 4–5 years [54, 58], significantly later than typical retinoblastoma presenting between 1 and 2 years of age [59], though there are published reports of cases diagnosed from 1 to 19 years [60]. An association has been shown with the *RB1* gene [57], though less than 5% have a known family history of retinoblastoma [58].

In children old enough to express symptoms, the most common presenting complaints include unilateral eye pain, floaters, and blurred vision [58]. The provider, patient, or family member may also notice injection or leukocoria [58]. Vitreous cell is the most common examination finding, reported in 79% of cases [58], followed by pseudohypopyon in 48% [58]. Intraocular pressure may be elevated in the affected eye [58]. Additional examination findings may include injections, cataracts, neovascularization of the iris, vitreous hemorrhages, or retinal detachments [54, 58].

Diffuse infiltrating retinoblastoma is often misdiagnosed as uveitis, especially when the presentation includes pain, conjunctival injection, and vitreous cells. Additional differential diagnoses include Coats disease, trauma, endophthalmitis, toxoplasmosis, or *Toxocara canis*, depending on presentation. The workup often begins with ultrasound, showing retinal thickening and calcification with hyper-reflective vitreous cells [54]. On computed tomography, approximately 67% have a detectable mass and 89% exhibit patchy calcification [54]. As with typical retinoblastoma, diagnostic vitreous sampling is contraindicated due to the risk of metastasis. Therefore, diagnosis is largely based on clinical findings and confirmed with pathology after enucleation.

Treatment for diffuse infiltrating retinoblastoma often includes enucleation. When metastasis is present, intensive systemic chemotherapy [61] may be required with agents including vincristine, etoposide, methotrexate, or carboplatin, though drug resistance is a significant concern.

5. Conclusions

Intraocular cells in any segment of the eye are most commonly a sign of inflammation but may be a harbinger of an insidious underlying malignancy. Ophthalmologists should be suspicious of an alternative diagnosis in patients presenting with signs and symptoms of uveitis who do not improve, or initially improve and then recur, with anti-inflammatory treatments. There are a slew of diagnostic tools available, many of which are relatively easy to perform, widely available, and noninvasive. The malignancies described above are considered masquerade syndromes commonly mistaken for uveitis, and their prompt diagnosis can be lifesaving.

Conflict of interest

The authors declare no conflict of interest.

Acronyms and abbreviations

OCT	optical coherence tomography
FAF	fundus autofluorescence
RPE	retinal pigment epithelium
PVRL	primary vitreoretinal lymphoma

DLBCL	diffuse large B-cell lymphoma
COMS	Collaborative Ocular Melanoma Study
HIV	Huma immunodeficiency virus
ELISA	enzyme-linked immunosorbent assay
PCR	polymerase chain reaction
FA	fundus autofluorescence
OD	oculus dexter
CT	computed tomography
MRI	magnetic resonance imaging
IL	interleukin

Author details

Teresa E. Fowler and Diego Espinosa-Heidmann*
Augusta University, Augusta, USA

*Address all correspondence to: deheidmann@augusta.edu

References

[1] Rothova A, Ooijman F, Kerkhoff F, Van der Lelij A, Lokhorst HM. Uveitis masquerade syndromes. Ophthalmology. 2001;**108**(2):386-399

[2] Chen PW, Murray TG, Salgaller ML, Ksander BR. Expression of MAGE genes in ocular melanoma cell lines. Journal of Immunotherapy. 1997;**20**(4):265-275

[3] Niederkorn JY, Wang S. REVIEW immunology of intraocular tumors. Ocular Immunology and Inflammation. 2005;**13**(1):105-110

[4] Fujimoto JG, Pitris C, Boppart SA, Brezinski ME. Optical coherence tomography: An emerging technology for biomedical imaging and optical biopsy. Neoplasia. 2000;**2**(1-2):9-25

[5] Shields CL, Mashayekhi A, Materin MA, Luo CK, Marr BP, Demirci H, et al. Optical coherence tomography of choroidal nevus in 120 patients. Retina. 2005;**25**(3):243-252

[6] Shields CL, Furuta M, Thangappan A, Nagori S, Mashayekhi A, Lally DR, et al. Metastasis of uveal melanoma millimeter-by-millimeter in 8033 consecutive eyes. Archives of Ophthalmology. 2009;**127**(8):989-998

[7] Coleman DJ, Lizzi FL, Jack RL. Ultrasonography of the Eye and Orbit. Philadelphia, PA: Lea & Febiger; 1977

[8] Kirmani M, Thomas E, Rao N, Laborde R. Intraocular reticulum cell sarcoma: Diagnosis by choroidal biopsy. British Journal of Ophthalmology. 1987;**71**(10):748-752

[9] Davis JL, Solomon D, Nussenblatt RB, Palestine AG, Chan C-C. Immunocytochemical staining of vitreous cells: Indications, techniques, and results. Ophthalmology. 1992;**99**(2):250-256

[10] Whitcup SM, de Smet MD, Rubin BI, Palestine AG, Martin DF, Burnier M Jr, et al. Intraocular lymphoma: Clinical and histopathologic diagnosis. Ophthalmology. 1993;**100**(9):1399-1406

[11] Zhuang Z, LeHoang P, Böni R, Zheng S, Nussenblatt RB, Chan C-C. Utility of microdissection and polymerase chain reaction for the detection of immunoglobulin gene rearrangement and translocation in primary intraocular lymphoma. Ophthalmology. 1998;**105**(9):1664-1669

[12] Ramsay A, Lightman S. Hypopyon uveitis. Survey of Ophthalmology. 2001;**46**(1):1-18

[13] Tyagi M, Govindhari V, Pappuru RR, Ambiya V. Bilateral hypopyon uveitis in chronic myeloid leukemia. Ocular Oncology and Pathology. 2018;**4**(1):12-15

[14] Kluin PM, Deckert M, Ferry JA. Primary diffuse large B-cell lymphoma of the CNS. In: Swerdlow SH, Campo E, Harris NL, Jaffe ES, Pileri SA, Stein H, et al., editors. World Health Organization Classification of Tumours of Haematopoietic and Lymphoid Tissues. Lyon: IARC Press; 2008. pp. 240-241

[15] Coupland SE, Anastassiou G, Bornfeld N, Hummel M, Stein H. Primary intraocular lymphoma of T-cell type: Report of a case and review of the literature. Graefe's Archive for Clinical and Experimental Ophthalmology. 2005;**243**(3):189-197

[16] Chan CC, Rubenstein JL, Coupland SE, Davis JL, Harbour JW, Johnston PB, et al. Primary vitreoretinal

lymphoma: A report from an international primary central nervous system lymphoma collaborative group symposium. The Oncologist. 2011;**16**(11):1589-1599

[17] Steffen J, Coupland SE, Smith JR. Primary vitreoretinal lymphoma in HIV infection. Ocular Immunology and Inflammation. 2021;**29**(3):621-627

[18] Coupland SE, Damato B. Understanding intraocular lymphomas. Clinical & Experimental Ophthalmology. 2008;**36**(6):564-578

[19] Lobo A, Larkin G, Clark BJ, Towler HM, Lightman S. Pseudo-hypopyon as the presenting feature in B-cell and T-cell intraocular lymphoma. Clinical & Experimental Ophthalmology. 2003;**31**(2):155-158

[20] Hormigo A, DeAngelis LM. Primary ocular lymphoma: Clinical features, diagnosis, and treatment. Clinical Lymphoma. 2003;**4**(1):22-29

[21] Cassoux N, Merle-Beral H, Leblond V, Bodaghi B, Miléa D, Gerber S, et al. Ocular and central nervous system lymphoma: Clinical features and diagnosis. Ocular Immunology and Inflammation. 2000;**8**(4):243-250

[22] Xu LT, Huang Y, Liao A, Anthony CL, Voloschin A, Yeh S. Multimodal diagnostic imaging in primary vitreoretinal lymphoma. International Journal of Retina and Vitreous. 2022;**8**(1):1-7

[23] Coupland SE. Analysis of intraocular biopsies. In: Current Concepts in Uveal Melanoma. Vol. 49. Karger: Basel; 2012

[24] Nirmal RM. Diagnosis of malignant lymphoma–An overview. Journal of Oral and Maxillofacial Pathology: JOMFP. 2020;**24**(2):195

[25] Bonzheim I, Giese S, Deuter C, Süsskind D, Zierhut M, Waizel M, et al. High frequency of MYD88 mutations in vitreoretinal B-cell lymphoma: A valuable tool to improve diagnostic yield of vitreous aspirates. Blood: The Journal of the American Society of Hematology. 2015;**126**(1):76-79

[26] Fishburne BC, Wilson DJ, Rosenbaum JT, Neuwelt EA. Intravitreal methotrexate as an adjunctive treatment of intraocular lymphoma. Archives of Ophthalmology. 1997;**115**(9):1152-1156

[27] Frenkel S, Hendler K, Siegal T, Shalom E, Peer J. Intravitreal methotrexate for treating vitreoretinal lymphoma: 10 years of experience. British Journal of Ophthalmology. 2008;**92**(3):383-388

[28] Hashida N, Ohguro N, Nishida K. Efficacy and complications of intravitreal rituximab injection for treating primary vitreoretinal lymphoma. Translational Vision Science & Technology. 2012;**1**(3):1-1

[29] Shields CL, Shields JA, Gross NE, Schwartz GP, Lally SE. Survey of 520 eyes with uveal metastases. Ophthalmology. 1997;**104**(8):1265-1276

[30] Aronow ME, Topham AK, Singh AD. Uveal melanoma: 5-year update on incidence, treatment, and survival (SEER 1973-2013). Ocular Oncology and Pathology. 2018;**4**(3):145-151

[31] Damato EM, Damato BE. Detection and time to treatment of uveal melanoma in the United Kingdom: An evaluation of 2384 patients. Ophthalmology. 2012;**119**(8):1582-1589

[32] Krantz BA, Dave N, Komatsubara KM, Marr BP, Carvajal RD. Uveal melanoma: Epidemiology, etiology, and treatment of primary disease. Clinical Ophthalmology (Auckland, NZ). 2017;**11**:279

[33] Shields CL, Kaliki S, Furuta M, Mashayekhi A, Shields JA. Clinical spectrum and prognosis of uveal melanoma based on age at presentation in 8,033 cases. Retina. 2012;**32**(7):1363-1372

[34] Egan KM, Seddon JM, Glynn RJ, Gragoudas ES, Albert DM. Epidemiologic aspects of uveal melanoma. Survey of Ophthalmology. 1988;**32**(4):239-251

[35] Coleman K, Baak J, Van Diest P, Mullaney J, Farrell M, Fenton M. Prognostic factors following enucleation of 111 uveal melanomas. British Journal of Ophthalmology. 1993;**77**(11):688-692

[36] Shields CL, Kaliki S, Cohen MN, Shields PW, Furuta M, Shields JA. Prognosis of uveal melanoma based on race in 8100 patients: The 2015 Doyne Lecture. Eye. 2015;**29**(8):1027-1035

[37] Andreoli MT, Mieler WF, Leiderman YI. Epidemiological trends in uveal melanoma. British Journal of Ophthalmology. 2015;**99**(11):1550-1553

[38] Feng L, Zhu J, Gao T, Li B, Yang Y. Uveal melanoma in the peripheral choroid masquerading as chronic uveitis. Optometry and Vision Science. 2014;**91**(9):e222

[39] Lentz K, Burns RP, Loeffler K, Feeney-Burns L, Berkelhammer J, Hook R. Uveitis caused by cytotoxic immune response to cutaneous malignant melanoma in swine: Destruction of uveal melanocytes during tumor regression. Investigative Ophthalmology & Visual Science. 1983;**24**(8):1063-1069

[40] Maat W, Ly LV, Jordanova ES, de Wolff-Rouendaal D, Schalij-Delfos NE, Jager MJ. Monosomy of chromosome 3 and an inflammatory phenotype occur together in uveal melanoma. Investigative Ophthalmology & Visual Science. 2008;**49**(2):505-510

[41] Coleman DJ, Silverman RH, Rondeau MJ, Boldt HC, Lloyd HO, Lizzi FL, et al. Noninvasive in vivo detection of prognostic indicators for high-risk uveal melanoma: Ultrasound parameter imaging. Ophthalmology. 2004;**111**(3):558-564

[42] Li L, Wang W-J, Chen R-J, Qian J, Luo C-Q, Zhang Y-J, et al. Fundus fluorescein angiography in metastatic choroidal carcinomas and differentiating metastatic choroidal carcinomas from primary choroidal melanomas. Chinese Journal of Ophthalmology. 2011;**47**(1):27-34

[43] McCannel TA. Fine-needle aspiration biopsy in the management of choroidal melanoma. Current Opinion in Ophthalmology. 2013;**24**(3):262-266

[44] Kujala E, Mäkitie T, Kivela T. Very long-term prognosis of patients with malignant uveal melanoma. Investigative Ophthalmology & Visual Science. 2003;**44**(11):4651-4659

[45] Diener-West M, Hawkins BS, Markowitz JA, Schachat AP. A review of mortality from choroidal melanoma: II. A meta-analysis of 5-year mortality rates following enucleation, 1966 through 1988. Archives of Ophthalmology. 1992;**110**(2):245-250

[46] Zimmerman LE, Mclean IW. An evaluation of enucleation in the management of uveal melanomas. American Journal of Ophthalmology. 1979;**87**(6):741-760

[47] Zimmerman LE, McLean I, Foster WD. Does enucleation of the eye containing a malignant melanoma prevent or accelerate the dissemination of tumour cells. British Journal of Ophthalmology. 1978;**62**(6):420-425

[48] The Collaborative Ocular Melanoma Study Group. The COMS randomized

trial of iodine 125 brachytherapy for choroidal melanoma, III: Initial mortality findings. Archives of Ophthalmology. 2001;**119**:969-982

[49] The Collaborative Ocular Melanoma Study Group. The Collaborative Ocular Melanoma Study (COMS) randomized trial of pre-enucleation radiation of large choroidal melanoma ii: Initial mortality findings COMS Report No. 10. American Journal of Ophthalmology. 1998;**125**(6):779-796

[50] Margo CE. The collaborative ocular melanoma study: An overview. Cancer Control. 2004;**11**(5):304-309

[51] Wang Z, Nabhan M, Schild SE, Stafford SL, Petersen IA, Foote RL, et al. Charged particle radiation therapy for uveal melanoma: A systematic review and meta-analysis. International Journal of Radiation Oncology, Biology, and Physics. 2013;**86**(1):18-26

[52] Shields CL, Mashayekhi A, Luo CK, Materin MA, Shields JA. Optical coherence tomography in children: Analysis of 44 eyes with intraocular tumors and simulating conditions. Journal of Pediatric Ophthalmology & Strabismus. 2004;**41**(6):338-344

[53] Foster BS, Mukai S. Intraocular retinoblastoma presenting as ocular and orbital inflammation. International Ophthalmology Clinics. 1996;**36**(1):153-160

[54] Shields CL, Ghassemi F, Tuncer S, Thangappan A, Shields JA. Clinical spectrum of diffuse infiltrating retinoblastoma in 34 consecutive eyes. Ophthalmology. 2008;**115**(12):2253-2258

[55] Kivelä T. The epidemiological challenge of the most frequent eye cancer: Retinoblastoma, an issue of birth and death. British Journal of Ophthalmology. 2009;**93**(9):1129-1131

[56] Kao L-Y. Diffuse infiltrating retinoblastoma: An inherited case. Retina. 2000;**20**(2):217-219

[57] Schedler KJ, Traine PG, Lohmann DR, Haritoglou C, Metz KA, Rodrigues EB. Hereditary diffuse infiltrating retinoblastoma. Ophthalmic Genetics. 2016;**37**(1):95-97

[58] Traine PG, Schedler KJ, Rodrigues EB. Clinical presentation and genetic paradigm of diffuse infiltrating retinoblastoma: A review. Ocular Oncology and Pathology. 2016;**2**(3):128-132

[59] Epstein JA, Shields CL, Shields JA. Trends in the management of retinoblastoma: Evaluation of 1,196 consecutive eyes during 1974 to 2001. Journal of Pediatric Ophthalmology & Strabismus. 2003;**40**(4):196-203

[60] Khanfir K, Chompret A, Frau E, Bloch-Michel E, Tursz T, Le Cesne A. An unusual variant of diffuse retinoblastoma in an adult. Acta Oncologica. 2008;**47**(5):973-974

[61] Dimaras H, Héon E, Budning A, Doyle JJ, Halliday W, Gallie BL, et al. Retinoblastoma CSF metastasis cured by multimodality chemotherapy without radiation. Ophthalmic Genetics. 2009;**30**(3):121-126